AGING WITH A DISABILITY

Aging with a Disability

Roberta B. Trieschmann, Ph.D.

Consulting Psychologist
Scottsdale, Arizona

DEMOS PUBLICATIONS
New York

This book is dedicated to
all the disabled people and their families
who have fought for
life, liberty, and the pursuit of happiness

Demos Publications, 156 Fifth Avenue, New York, New York 10010

Made in the United States of America

Great care has been taken to maintain the accuracy of the information contained in this volume. However, Dr. Roberta B. Trieschmann and Demos Publications cannot be held responsible for errors or for any consequences arising from the use of the information contained herein.

ISBN: 0-939957-01-9

LC: 86-72100

Preface

Prior to World War II, individuals with physical disabilities were not very visible in American society; a majority did not survive the acute injury or illness, and those who did were not usually found in the mainstream of American life. However, the development of the sulfanilamides and antibiotics in the 1930s and 1940s changed the survival statistics so that by the end of World War II we had a sizable and visible population of persons with major physical disabilities incurred during active military duty. The polio epidemics of the 1940s and 1950s added an additional civilian population of persons with disability, and now both of these groups are aging—aging with a physical disability.

The Spinal Cord Research Foundation (SCRF) of the Paralyzed Veterans of America (PVA) has been aware of the problems occurring in the lives of people with major long-term physical disabilities and therefore has been interested in sponsoring research to provide answers to questions relevant to this topic. After soliciting research proposals on this issue, it became obvious to the SCRF that no consensus existed as to the nature of the aging problem and the questions that needed to be answered. This book developed from a research contract awarded to this author by SCRF to identify what we know and do not know about the issues of aging with a major disability so that a strategy for future research could be developed. The methodology for this project included a review of the scientific literature and personal unstructured interviews with persons who have long-term disability, with their families, and with rehabilitation professionals. It is of interest to note that the majority of the professional literature is oriented to acute illness and injury, and long-term disability is often defined as 18 months to 5 years after onset. As a result, it seems clear that those with disabilities of 20 or more years are indeed a forgotten population for professionals.

No attempt has been made to review the massive amount of literature on the topic of gerontology in general; this is beyond the scope of this book. However, the body of this text repeatedly emphasizes the need to compare the incidence of problems in the aging disabled population with that found in the aging "nondisabled" population so that we do not erroneously overestimate or overinterpret the scope or depth of difficulties experienced by the disabled group. This is the issue of base rates—the average frequency of occurrence of an event in the population at large—which is discussed in Chapter 4.

Rehabilitation professionals without physical disabilities are not the repository of all knowledge about life with a disability. Rather, the true experts are those who have survived with the residuals of a major illness or injury for 30,

40, or 50 years, and this author has placed great emphasis on gaining information from these individuals. As a result, a series of personal interviews was held with disabled individuals and family members in a variety of locations around the United States. Both civilians and veterans were interviewed; all were telephoned personally by this author, the purpose of the project explained, and a request for an interview made. No one refused. The interviews lasted from two to six hours and all were conducted face-to-face. The cities in which these people reside have been deliberately omitted in order to ensure anonymity of the individuals and the confidentiality of the information revealed. No attempt was made to ensure the statistical representativeness of the sample, since the purpose of the interviews was to elicit ideas, not to document incidence of problems. That is a task for future research.

At this point, it should be noted that some of the ideas and opinions presented in this book may be controversial. However, they represent those of the author and her informants and do not necessarily represent those of any organizations that have provided financial support to the author during the research or the writing of this book.

This work should be useful to physicians, psychologists, social workers, nurses, physical and occupational therapists, policymakers, legislators, researchers, teachers, and all of us who are aging and plan to do so in the future. Hopefully, it will serve to stimulate new research and form the basis for enlightened clinical practice and social legislation. But most of all I am concerned that this work provide some measure of hope and reassurance to all people who are aging and who have physical disabilities: hope that changes can and will be made; reassurance that you are not alone. There are many people who do care what happens to you.

R.B.T.

Acknowledgments

The inspiration for this book was provided by the Spinal Cord Research Foundation (SCRF) of the Paralyzed Veterans of America (PVA) who awarded a research contract to the author to identify what we know and do not know about aging with a physical disability. I would like to thank the Board of Trustees of SCRF for this support, and Lynn Phillips, Research Director, and Thomas Stripling, Senior Associate Research Director, for their invaluable assistance and encouragement throughout the entire project.

Early into the research, however, it became exceedingly clear that one could not discuss the concept of aging outside of the context of how we treat aging people in the United States, especially the type of health care services that we do and do not provide to ease their burdens. Thus, an essential feature of this document is a discussion of our health care delivery system in regards to its approach to those who are aging and disabled. Many of these ideas have been evolving in my work for many years, but they became much more focused over the last four years. Part of this study into health care delivery was sponsored by a Mary E. Switzer Senior Research Fellowship from the National Institute for Handicapped Research (NIHR), Office of Special Education and Rehabilitation Services, Department of Education, for which I am very grateful. I would like to thank J. Paul Thomas, Ph.D., my project officer during the fellowship, and Douglas Fenderson, Ph.D., past Director of NIHR.

Many people with long-term disabilities and their families and many health care professionals have freely and frankly offered their observations and opinions on this topic. Without them, the document would have very limited value. In order to protect the anonymity of those who revealed confidential information, I will not specifically identify names. You all know who you are and I thank you.

These are some names that can be and should be mentioned. Ernest Bors, M.D., urologist and paraplegist extraordinaire, was particularly helpful in outlining the variety of medical issues that need to be considered in research of this type. George W. Hohmann, Ph.D., has been a valued colleague for many years and was particularly helpful during the idea-generating and writing phases of this research. Several individuals agreed to review the manuscript for me; among these are: Lynn Phillips; George W. Hohmann; Angelo Nicosia, Hospital Liaison Director, Eastern PVA; Ellen Pilcher, M.A., Independent Living Specialist, Arizona Bridge to Independent Living; William A. Spencer, M.D., President of the Texas Institute for Rehabilitation and Research and Professor and Chairman of Rehabilitation Medicine, Baylor College of Medicine; and

Judith K. Polk, educated layperson. To each of these individuals my deep thanks for giving me their time and invaluable feedback on a topic that is important to all of us.

However, the real "angel" of this endeavor is my husband, A. Clyde Flackbert, Ph.D., who has, throughout our marriage, provided the ideal atmosphere for some of my most creative professional work.

Contents

1

Introduction

Aging is synonymous with living; it is a process that begins at birth and evolves across the life span. Actually, aging is the process of adjusting to a constantly changing internal and external environment, and, as a result, there is no definable beginning point for being "aged." Rather, this concept creeps into our awareness after we make a series of adjustments to accommodate the realization that we cannot do as many of the things we did when we were younger. Usually the change is subtle, evolving over many years so that "normal aging" results in the gradual reduction in scope and intensity of our activities. Sometimes the change is sudden, however, if we experience a major disability. Thus, many older people find that the miracles of modern medicine provide them with the opportunity to continue to live but with a sudden alteration of many dimensions of their lives.

There is another population, however, that has been overlooked: those who experienced a major disability in the earlier years of their lives, who have adjusted to the altered lifestyle, and who are now experiencing another decline in scope and intensity of activities. Thus, the issue of aging with a disability is a new problem for western societies, one that has caught our health care system by surprise. Currently, individuals who have lived with spinal injury, polio, and other disabilities for 30, 40, and 50 years are arriving in physicians' offices with a variety of complaints that the physicians have not been taught to handle. For example, spinal injury had been viewed as a static disability, with the major medical interventions occurring in the first several years after disability onset. Thus, the medical literature concentrates on the management of acute spinal injury and the initial rehabilitation of the person in preparation for discharge to his or her home and community. Medical management of these individuals has been the province of a few specialities, primarily those of physiatry (physical medicine and rehabilitation), orthopedic surgery, neurosurgery, and urology. Therefore, few other physicians are knowledgable about the problems that can occur in those with this disability. Polio has been viewed as an infectious disease that has been virtually eradicated in western countries and, thus, is not even mentioned today in medical schools except in an historical context. As a result, most of the physicians in practice today have never worked with acute poliomyelitis and, consequently, have little familiarity with the types of residual deficits and complications with which post-polio persons live. Other individuals with multiple sclerosis, cerebral palsy, spina bifida—all of whom have lived a large part of their lives with a physical disability—are aging and experiencing difficulties after 20 or 30 years with the impairment. Moreover, many people are acquiring a physical disability in the later years of life, and the number of these individuals is growing with each new advance in medical technology.

Forty years ago, there were very few people with major disabilities who were visible in their communities, partly because they did not survive very long after onset of the disease and partly because they were not accepted readily by society. Those who lived tended to stay in the home with little expectation that a "normal" life was possible or perhaps even "proper."

However, in the aftermath of World War II, the developed nations were confronted with a large number of men with disabilities, and the sheer numbers of these individuals attracted attention. Furthermore, the development of the sulfanilamides and antibiotics produced miraculous survival rates because people were no longer dying as readily of the initial complications, such as infection. In addition, the polio epidemics of the 1940s and 1950s added thousands of persons with disabilities to the number who had survived World War II, and, thus, the field of rehabilitation was born with the avowed purpose of teaching individuals to work around the disability in order to become as independent and self-sufficient as possible. Return to a fairly normal life began to seem possible, and, by their sheer numbers, these individuals could not be hidden in the back bedrooms anymore. In fact, this group refused to do so. The young men disabled during the Second World War were heroes, of course, and our polio survivors were mostly young, energetic, and vital people.

As a result, the field of rehabilitation has grown spectacularly in the last 40 years, and most physically disabled people can count on an almost normal life span, given the specifics of their disability and life circumstances. But now, as the ultimate sign of success in this field, individuals with disabilities are aging; they are experiencing a constellation of problems that may be a combination of "normal" aging and problems unique to life with a specific disability. Unfortunately, most professionals have little understanding of the scope of the aging and disability problem, little conception of the types of questions that need to be researched, little knowledge of how to handle the problems these people present for treatment.

Often one thinks of aging as strictly a biological or organic change in function. However, in the course of research for this book, it became clear that *the biological changes experienced by persons who are aging are relevant—are potentially problematical—not only because of discomfort but because of the adaptations required in personal lifestyle and the additional environmental supports needed to compensate for altered or declining biological function.* The search for the fountain of youth has yielded meager results (despite the entreaties of Madison Avenue for this or that product), and the miracles of modern medicine have failed to extend life beyond the fourscore of earlier years (changes in average life expectancy are mostly the result of reduced infant mortality, vaccination, and improved public sanitation and nutrition), and consequently we are all faced with the fact that certain biological functions decline with age and these cannot be easily "fixed" or prevented.

Thus, *the essential problem of aging is not only how to treat declining biological–organic function but also how to adapt the environment to allow the person to be as functional as possible—to work around or compensate for the altered biological function.* Certainly, if a biological problem can be ameliorated, wonderful. Go for it. But when it cannot be remedied or fixed, it is shortsighted and wrong to assume that nothing can be done. Consequently, a strictly medical, biological–organic approach to aging (whether disabled or "nondisabled") is inappropriate. Rather, a systems approach to interventions is the strategy most suited to meet the challenges of the problem.

We talk about a health care system in the United States, but actually we are evolving toward a sickness treatment business establishment despite the good intentions and efforts of some very caring professionals. Because aging is not strictly a medical problem, and because aging is not always necessarily a sickness that can be treated, a sickness treatment system, designed to attend mostly to biological–organic dysfunctions, is the worst of all possible approaches to the complex biopsychosocial, environmental problem of aging.

In the research for this book on aging with a disability, it became clear that little attention had been given to this topic by the scientific community. Defining the topics for the computerized literature search immediately presented some unexpected problems. The key words "aging with disability" produced little of use. After trying many combinations of key words, it became obvious that the professional literature on the topic was minimal to nonexistent. Thus, a computerized literature search using the key word "spinal diseases" was conducted with the intention of ferreting out any articles that may even indirectly allude to older persons with disability. Other articles and books relevant to the topic had to be identified through bibliographic searches and discussions with other knowledgable professionals.

The idea of conducting one-on-one interviews came about when the original plan of holding consumer conferences in several key cities in the United States had to be abandoned because only two couples of the 22 expected showed up for the first conference. They explicitly stated that valid information can only be gained through personal interviews because the very process of surviving and overcoming the barriers to the disabled has taught each of them to "look good," "act invulnerable," and "maintain face" in front of others, especially in front of those without disabilities. These two spinal-injured men and their wives had a powerful impact on the research process because they had the courage to come and tell me that my plan would not work and then they opened up to me for six hours and set the stage for all further interviews. These two men, Robert Moss and Sandy Weinzimer, passed away in less than a year after that interview, but their spirit and that of their wives live on in this book.

Consequently, it was decided to hold personal interviews with disabled individuals and family members throughout the United States. The interviews were facilitated via contacts made through the network of professionals and persons with disabilities known to the author. All interviewees had been disabled at least 30 years and were experiencing some life changes associated with aging. (It is interesting to note that aging actually relates to the duration of the disability rather than chronological age. Thus, it appears that after 20 or more years with a disability a person *may* begin to experience some changes in function regardless of one's calendar age. Consequently, *some* individuals who acquired polio in their early childhood may experience "aging" problems in their 30s.)

This book establishes a conceptual framework for the discussion of aging with a disability. The concept of health or adjustment is defined as the balance achieved among three major influences in life: psychosocial (P), biological–organic (O), and environmental (E). Behavior, health, or adjustment (B) is the interactive result of these three influences, i.e., $B = f(P,O,E)$. Aging is viewed as a change in the balance, often the result of the alteration of biological–organic (O) function, which then has an impact on the psychosocial (P) and environmental (E) influences in life. Interventions need to be directed not only at the biological–organic (O) problem, but most particularly at restoring the balance in the psychosocial (P) and environmental (E) realms of life. Thus, it becomes necessary to discuss the concept of sickness treatment versus health care in regard to this concept of aging in order to define the problems and establish the questions for future research.

This conceptualization of the process of aging has broad utility. *This book focuses on those with major physical disabilities, but the concepts are equally applicable to all other aging people, those without disabilities and those with head injury or developmental or emotional impairments.* It is a major premise of this book that the labeling of disabled and "nondisabled" is an artificial distinction—an arbitrary division of a continuum into two parts. Physical function is only a matter of degree as are cognitive clarity and emotional balance, all of these being fluctuating phenomena in any of our lives. Thus, we consider the terms disabled and "nondisabled" to be verbal conveniences only.

Another premise of this book is that it is inappropriate to use the term "patients" to refer generically to those with disabilities. The *Random House Dictionary* defines "patient" as a person undergoing medical or surgical treatment and the synonym given is "invalid." Since the status of "patient" within most medical centers is one of relative powerlessness, it reinforces negative attitudes to apply this term to those with impairments when they are not formally seeking services from the health care system. Also, as we move toward a more enlightened concept of health care, one of a partnership between the individual and professional, it is helpful to use terms reflective of mutual respect for each other's knowledge and responsibility in the health care process. Therefore, let us develop the habit of using the terms "persons" or "individuals" at all times.

The demographic projections of the United States indicate that those aged 65 years or older will constitute an increasing percentage of the population over the next decades. As these individuals age, they too will experience problems when altered biological–organic (O) function tips the health and adjustment balance. This will place stress on the psychological realm of function (P) and often will require additional environmental support services (E) in order to keep people functioning satisfactorily in their own homes. Therefore, the principles discussed in this book apply to the lives of all of us, those of us who are currently in the upper decades of life and those of us who plan to get there.

Consequently, in this book we review what we know and do not know about the process of aging with a disability. Because each human is a unique system, a psychological, biological–organic, environmental system, there will be a varying combination of these variables influencing each of our lives, as is illustrated by the biographies of people with disabilities presented in Chapter 2. These people have great personal strength, but, as will become apparent, personal will is not always sufficient in cases of major disability. Popular lore suggests that, if you have the "right stuff," you can prevail and overcome any difficulty. Yet, the physical disability in combination with the environment present a handicap that penalizes the disabled person in comparison to the "nondisabled" person. Moreover, this penalty increases with age and that becomes the focus of the remainder of this book.

As a result, this book has been written for all of us—all of us are aging, all of us experience a decline in energy and altered physical function over time. For some, however, this very natural process is superimposed on other impairments that have imposed a physical, emotional, and financial penalty on daily life. Unfortunately for these people with major physical disabilities, the process of aging seems to increase the amount of the penalty.

2

The Fight for Life, Liberty, and the Pursuit of Happiness

The fight for the right to life, liberty, and the pursuit of happiness has been a major theme in the history of the human race, and in our century the struggles of certain groups stand out from the rest. In the last 50 years, we have experienced a world war against totalitarianism, the Jews and Palestinians fight for the right to a homeland, and numerous other groups fight for religious and economic freedoms. Within the United States, black Americans have fought for civil rights, women still seek equal rights, and persons with major physical disabilities still fight for freedom and equality. They have survived what had been certain death, lived comfortable and not so comfortable lives outside of a hospital, sought economic freedom, and now are experiencing the problems of aging in addition to the daily travail of living with a physical disability. We know little about the aging and disability process because this group has and will serve as pioneers throughout their lives. They taught us how to live with disability and now they will teach us how to age and die with disability. However, in order to understand the issues of aging in this group, we need to know what they have experienced in the 30, 40, and 50 years that they have lived with their disabilities because it has been a fight for life, liberty, and the pursuit of happiness on their own terms. They are the *pioneers*; they are the *survivors*, and this totally shapes their perception of aging and their strategies for coping with it. Thus, the stories of eight people will be presented to illustrate how various combinations of psychosocial (P), biological–organic (O), and environmental (E) resources shape the process of living with the disability and the dimensions of the aging process.

FRANK
The World War II Veteran

It was the "good war," but it was a "no win" situation according to the average serviceman. In the autumn of 1942 at the age of 19, Frank enlisted in the

6

army and was assigned to the Army Specialized Training Program (ASTP) at Ohio State University in the engineering program even though English Literature had been his avowed interest. The army told him that in one and a half years he would obtain a Bachelor of Science degree by taking 40 hours of class a week; unfortunately, without warning, the program was terminated in March 1944 as the preparations for D-Day escalated. The army needed men to fight in the foxholes, lots of men, and the personal reaction of "but they can't do this to me" was replaced by anxious resignation. This was World War II. You did not enlist for two years and then have the choice of re-enlisting or going home; you were in for the duration of the war and there was no way out. Well, there was actually: you went crazy (or self-inflicted a wound); you were injured in combat; you were killed; or the war was over. In November 1944, one of the first three happened to the average soldier within six weeks. One day after Frank was wounded, his platoon (40 men), which had been at full strength, was reduced to four men.

On the Maginot-Siegfried Line, it was November 29, 1944. As a runner, Frank crawled on his belly across an open field carrying a colored panel to a German bunker to identify it for the fighter-bombers. On the return trip, he was shot in the back at T9-10 (in the thoracic level of the spine, at the 9th and 10th vertebrae). There was bombing and shooting all around him, but Frank was exhilarated and relieved, "I'm wounded and not dead. I'm out! I'm alive." However, after lying there for two hours, he noticed that he was bleeding heavily, couldn't move his legs, and then, only then, the thought occurred to him that he might die. In a panic, he started wondering how a person died, because if he could figure this out maybe he could stop this from happening. Finally, the medics got to him and he entered a series of medic stations and field hospitals in Belgium until he could be transferred to England. During this time he had a terrible pain in his back whenever he was moved, a tube was inserted into his bladder that he was told to watch without knowing why, and his x-ray films, hanging on a line above his cot, revealed the location of the bullet in his back. The neurosurgeon told him that he had a fifty-fifty chance of living whether or not the bullet was removed, so Frank told him to take it out. After surgery, he was transferred to a general hospital on a sheet of plywood to keep his back straight and then placed on his back in bed and never turned. When he arrived in England seven days later, he had been in and out of consciousness and generally pretty sick. One dream recurred incessantly. Frank was in an underground cavern somewhere between life and death, but it was muddy like a foxhole. Mud was dripping from the ceiling and occasionally a soldier's body would drop through; these were dead bodies. Again and again he had the same nightmare and awoke screaming. Finally, in one recurrence of the dream, he got some timbers to brace up the ceiling and cover it to stop the leaks, to stop those bodies from dropping through. At that point he woke up, told the nurses that he would be OK now, and asked for food. He never had the dream again.

For the next year and a half, the nurses and volunteers were the heroines of the story because Frank almost never saw a physician. Having survived the initial crisis, he found himself in an American army hospital in Southhampton, England, and was introduced to Mildred Ellis, army nurse extraordinaire. Back on regular food, Frank had his first bowel movement, in bed, which mortified him terribly. She cleaned him up and explained about the lack of bowel and bladder control, what the catheter was for, and why he should make sure it was always draining freely. She insisted that he be turned every several hours (through luck and good protoplasm he did not have a pressure sore), but any movement sent a burning pain along his spine. Thus, some royal battles ensued. Mildred insisted that he would be turned; Frank insisted that he would not. Finally, Mildred got anry and rolled to his bedside another paraplegic with a massive, hideous pressure sore on his buttocks from unrelieved pressure on that area. Frank was horrified and sickened at the sight. She gave him a mirror and told him to check his bottom constantly. "Take charge of your own life, young man. No one will do it for you. If you rely on others, you will surely die." From that time there were no more battles about turning. At Christmas, Frank wrote to his sister that he was temporarily paralyzed but OK. He hoped he'd get well soon but not soon enough to be sent to the Pacific before the war ended. After the first of the year, spasticity (involuntary muscle movement) started in his legs, and he began to get reflex erections which to him were a sign of impending recovery. But there were the bladder infections, one after another, that kept him constantly nauseated, feverish, and miserable.

In February, he was transferred to the United States and arrived at Halloran Army Hospital on Staten Island to find such overcrowding that he was relegated to a cot in the hallway. The nurses were overworked so Frank would snag a passing Grey Lady volunteer to help him turn. They always protested that they were not allowed to touch patients, but he would insist and they relented. They always gave him the care that he needed even though it was against the rules. From Halloran, he traveled by train in March 1945 to Bushnell Army Hospital in Brigham City, Utah. This was a neurological and amputee center and he was the fourth person with spinal cord injury (SCI) to arrive. Eventually there would be 60.

After arrival at Bushnell, the reality of his situation began to set in. Suspecting that the paralysis might be permanent, he started to get depressed. This is not surprising, since the attitude at the hospital was one of deliberate neglect while waiting for these men with spinal injury to die. After all, prior to World War II, the death rate from spinal injury was as high as 80% during the acute phase (Carroll, 1970). The nurses and volunteers were wonderful women, but there were too few of them to handle all the care; thus, army and civilian orderlies were brought in, many of whom were far below normal intelligence, some of whom were mean. These orderlies used no sterile technique when irrigating the bladder catheters or changing the drainage systems, so that one man's bladder infection was transmitted to the next, and thus, they were never free of bladder infections and always sick. By June, Frank expected to die. He had shrunk from 210 to 96 pounds. The SCI men spent every day, all day, in bed except for once a week when their turn came to use one of the two huge cane-backed wheelchairs allotted to the spinal injury ward. Frank protested to Colonel "X," the army physician in charge of the ward, that two wheelchairs for 60 men was ridiculous. Colonel "X" responded that the army couldn't afford to buy wheelchairs for a bunch of guys with spinal injuries. "You don't need wheelchairs because you are going to die and there is not a thing that I can do to prevent that."

When the war ended, the men really became depressed because they had had legitimacy as long as the war lasted. Now they were refuse and expected to be dumped into a local Veterans Administration (VA) hospital near their hometown. Nothing happened, however, and the warehousing of the spinal injured continued. During that time, Frank used his ingenuity and learned to turn himself in bed. Also, he decided to use his army private's pay to purchase his own wheelchair for $250 so that he could get out of bed whenever he wanted.

In November 1945, the Surgeon General planned to make an inspection of Bushnell Army Hospital so Colonel "X" ordered clean sheets to be placed across each bed and all of the wheels on the beds to face in a uniform direction. Tidal drainage systems for bladder management were hung by each bed with the tube running under the sheet. However, the system was never connected to collect urine, since it would be a waste of time to have to clean all of that apparatus for men who would die anyway. When the Surgeon General, accompanied by Colonel "X," visited the ward, Lieutenant A (head nurse of the spinal injury unit) remained seated in her office, feet up on the desk, smoking a cigarette. The Surgeon General was surprised at such behavior from a nurse and asked her what was going on. She replied, "I refuse to participate in this charade of making these fellows look nice for inspection while actually allowing them to lie there in shit and waiting for them to die. Surely something can be done to make their lives better." Lieutenant A was court-marshalled by the hospital commandant and assigned to the boondocks; Colonel "X" was relieved of his command, and a young eager physician was sent in as his replacement. This young man called a meeting of the spinal injury group and told them that there was a physician at an army hospital in Modesto, California, a Dr. Bors, who was doing some new things for SCI and that he planned to visit him in order to learn what he could. Six weeks later he returned. The SCI men were now expected to be out of bed daily; they received wheelchairs to use; physical therapy equipment was obtained for muscle strengthing, transfers, and ambulation training if possible. Bowel and bladder programs with sterile technique were initiated, and a car with hand controls was obtained for driver education. This was a remarkable and exciting reversal, like day following night. They became independent, took trips out of the hospital, went to restaurants, participated in volleyball and swimming, and began to enjoy life after a year of waiting to die. The volunteers invited them into their homes and arranged for them to meet a spinal-injured member of their community. Since they all expected to die and never leave the hospital, this was their first evidence that one might indeed survive a spinal injury.

In the winter of 1945-46, the government initiated a plan to close the army hospitals by sending the men home, if possible, or, in the case of spinal injury and other severe disabilities, to the VA hospital nearest their hometown. But the men with SCI protested. It never occurred to them that they could go home to live; they would rather stick together than be the only SCI in the local VA even if it was possible to be near their families. At this point, there was a greater sense of community and "normality" with other SCIs than with their loved ones, to whom they were "deviant." Thus, they formed an organization to lobby for SCI centers in the VA hospitals and for provisions in proposed legislation to allow GI amputees to buy cars with hand controls. This informal organization at Bushnell was the forerunner of the current Paralyzed Veterans of America.

Bushnell closed in June 1946. There would be six VA SCI Centers initially, but all of the group from Bushnell were sent to Birmingham VA Hospital in Van Nuys, California (later to become the Long Beach VA), with Dr. Ernest Bors as physician in charge of the SCI Center. In the summer of 1946, there were 180 men with SCI there: 160 with paraplegia and only 20 with quadriplegia! They had been discharged from the military, had money to spend from their disability compensations, and a $1600 allotment to buy a car. This, however, was enough only to purchase a Chevrolet or Ford with a manual transmission, not amenable to hand controls. But with the shortage of cars for the general public after World War II, the men had no trouble selling the Chevy or Ford at a premium, allowing them to buy an Oldsmobile with automatic transmission. Thus in 1946, there were 180 Oldmobiles and a few Cadillacs parked outside of the Birmingham VA Hospital and it was a time of unbridled hedonism. They were alive; they were young; they had money; and they were in southern California with palm trees, sunshine, and beautiful women. At that time, Dr. Bors estimated that they might live as long as five years so they set about raising some hell with no consequences to pay. It was literally a matter of "eat, drink, and be merry, for tomorrow we may die." And quite a few of them did. Bladder and kidney infections took their toll, as did respiratory infections, especially among those with quadriplegia.

There was ambivalence in the general public about these men with SCI. They were heroes after all and nothing was too good for "our boys"...as long as they stayed out of sight. Frank and his buddies were often refused seats in restaurants because their presence would be too depressing to the other customers. Yet, there were some signs of enlightenment. UCLA agreed to accept four of the SCI group from the Birmingham VA in the undergraduate program; Frank was one of the four. They lived in the hospital, went to the campus for classes, and were allowed to take two courses the first semester. If they had trouble gaining access to certain buildings, a group called the CAL-VETS would meet them and carry them and wheelchairs up the stairs to their classes. The second semester, February 1947, Frank moved into a minimally wheelchair-adapted apartment on campus, took three courses, and got As in them. Meanwhile many of the fellows were beginning to get married and where they would live became the issue. Because of the reluctance of the community to accept disabled people and a lack of accessible housing, the idea of "Vet-Ville" gained momentum. A piece of land would be obtained in the San Fernando Valley region of Los Angeles on which would be built accessible housing, accessible shops and services, and some type of employment for the men. However, the PL 702 Housing legislation, which passed in 1948, gave veterans a $10,000 grant, plus up to a $10,000 GI loan to purchase a house. Thus, the idea of "Vet-Ville," segregated living for persons with disabilities, never got past the concept stage as the newly married men with spinal injury bought GI-financed homes in regular neighborhoods and resumed normal lives.

Frank, along with most of the fellows, staunchly maintained the attitude of "live today, for tomorrow I may die," but gradually some of the attitudes learned during the depression of the 1930s crept back into their consciousness. They started to get the message that they might live a while and the great bonanza of the government disability compensation, the car, the house, and the medical benefits might all disappear. No one expected the benefits to continue, and, thus, many of them started to think about what work they could do to earn a living. At this point, Frank settled down and took college seriously enough to earn a bachelor's, masters, and doctorate in clinical psychology. In 1948, he married a college classmate, Eleanor, but not without reservations on the part of his family. Frank was warned that she would never stick with him, the underlying message being, "Why would a woman settle for a paraplegic? After all, eventually she'll want a (real) man." Her family wasn't against the marriage, but since she had an inheritance of $30,000 (a magnificent sum in 1948), the subtle message was, "Why do you want to marry him? You don't need the money." These reactions were not unique but characterized the responses many of the SCI men and their women received from family and friends, because the notion that a person with a severe physical disability could lead a "normal" life just was not deemed reasonable. Money was a factor in a few of the marriages, but these did not last very long. Most of the marriages were based on love, loyalty, trust, sharing: all of the traditional virtues that characterize successful marriages. And indeed the marriages were successful as documented by El Ghatit and Hanson (1975, 1976).

Frank and Eleanor decided to adopt children, again an unheard-of notion, according to adoption agencies. These agencies had eliminated from consideration anyone who had a physical defect, the underlying message being that, if a father or mother was physically disabled, the child would grow up to be psychologically maladjusted. After meeting the minimal requirement for consideration, marriage of two years' duration, Eleanor began calling or visiting all of the adoption agencies in the Los Angeles region asking for application forms.

However, they would not even give her the forms, much less interview them as a couple, because of the physical defect rule. She called or visited these agencies every three months until 1953, when one prominent agency advised her that the reason that she and her husband would not be considered was that recent research indicated that spinal-injured men did not live very long. Certainly, they could not place a child in such a home. These data were contained in the thesis of the newly appointed director of the agency. Perceiving a potential loophole, Frank talked with Dr. Bors, who promptly called the director and asked her how she could be so definitive on longevity in spinal injury when he himself did not have such data. Well, she backed down and by the end of the conversation she had agreed to meet with Frank and Eleanor for an interview, a major victory in itself.

Frank and Eleanor went to the agency to meet the director, who insisted that the rules did not allow her to place children in families in which one party was an amputee, much less someone with a spinal injury. But they persisted and asked for a home study to evalute their assets and liabilities, realizing that the physical disability would be considered a liability. They pleaded that it was only fair to judge the entire family situation and then make a decision rather than prejudging them only on the basis of the disability. She relented, and since this was such an unprecedented undertaking, she decided to do the home study herself rather than delegate it to one of her staff. After many months of paperwork, interviews, and home visits, the director admitted that her experience in this case had forced the agency to reconsider all of the standards by which they judged homes and families. While her staff was not enthusiastic about the idea, she would place a child with them and would consider applications for adoption from other families with physical disability. Thus, Frank and Eleanor adopted a boy and a girl, who have now completed their doctorates and are each happily married.

The black market in babies was another route that Frank and Eleanor had considered as did a number of other people with physical disabilities. Essentially this amounted to paying money to a private party to obtain a child for adoption. This process was and still is laden with difficulties and, thus, they chose to avoid this avenue, although they did seriously consider it as an alternative at one point.

Some spinal-injured men sired their own children, but these men usually had incomplete spinal injuries. Artificial insemination was another alternative; however, the legal parenthood of such children had not been established at that time, and as a result, couples choosing this option would use a mixture of donor sperm and the husband's sperm.

In 1945, Frank was told that he would die soon and that life for him would consist of hospitalization and invalidism. It is interesting to examine the word "invalid." The *Random House Dictionary* defines invalid, a noun, as an "infirm or sickly person; a person who is too sick, weak, or old to care for himself; a person disabled by sickness or old age, i.e., a hopeless invalid." Invalid, as an adjective, is defined as "not valid; without force or foundation; indefensible; deficient in substance or cogency; weak, void or without legal force." These were the concepts that shaped the reality of the existence of persons with disabilities in the 1930s, 1940s, and 1950s, perhaps even today.

The connotation of "invalid" conveyed a set of expectations for performance sent by society to the person, and because quite realistically few severely disabled persons survived in those days, the newly disabled person had no information to the contrary, no success stories to point to, no role models. They were "deviant" in comparison to the rest of society, which is why the SCI veterans initially lobbied to stay together. But as life continued, when they did not die, as they began to participate in the natural activities of life, such as having fun, being independent, dating, and getting married, they gradually returned to the mainstream of life without necessarily planning to do so. And they learned from one another.

Each person's story is as innovative and courageous as Frank's. They shared information, tried different aspects of living, gave feedback and new ideas to each other. The medical profession was dedicated to doing the best that it could but it was as unknowing about the future of those with spinal injury as those living with it. Initially when they got to the Birmingham VA Hospital, Dr. Bors estimated that they had five years to live. When Frank got married in 1948, he asked Dr. Bors about life expectancy and the estimate then was 10–15 years. When Frank and Eleanor wanted to adopt children, life expectancy was placed at another 20 years.

The initial message of imminent death strongly influenced this group so that they have never taken life for granted. However, the natural process of living gradually propelled these men into all of the normal activities of life: finding jobs, going to school, marrying, having children. All of these events sent a message of normality. But of equal if not more importance, the government sponsorship of school, cars, housing, and disability compensation was reaffirming and sent a message of validity to counteract the general societal expectation of invalidity.

Frank and Eleanor will celebrate their 38th wedding anniversary in 1986. He served as psychologist and chief psychologist within the VA system and retired after 25 years to become a Professor of Psychology at a state university. Mildred Ellis, army nurse extraordinaire, did her job well; he has never had a pressure sore after 42 years in a wheelchair. After a lifetime of good health (except for hypertension), medical problems have occurred recently. A rectal fistula and abscess involved six months' hospitalization and surgical repair in 1982-83, leaving him with a colostomy and scar tissue on his buttocks, now making them more vulnerable to pressure sores. However, Frank's usual impeccable self-care has prevented any skin problems, and he is now in good health again. The extended hospitalization and recovery period prompted him to retire from the university, but he was awarded emeritus status soon after retirement. Although not officially involved in many professional activities, he remains consultant emeritus to all those who work in the professions concerned with physical disability.

Since Frank has a service-connected disability, he receives disability compensation from the VA of $40,000 a year, tax free, and receives a retirement pension from the VA after 25 years of full-time work. This pension is taxable. Upon his death, his service-connected disability compensation ceases, but Eleanor will receive Dependent Indemnity Compensation (DIC) of $4,800 a year plus 55% of his work pension. All of his medical expenses are paid by the VA, and, as a service-connected disabled veteran, he receives top priority for care over nonservice-connected disabled veterans. They own their own home and have invested wisely but are not rich. Eleanor should have ample money to live on upon his death because of his work pension, her work pension, and the financial cushion which the VA disability compensation has provided during Frank's life.

Would he do it over again, live life as a paraplegic in exchange for the financial security? No. There is no amount of money that would prompt him to live as a disabled person again. One does not choose to have a disability, but if it happens, most people make the best of the situation. Therefore, Frank reiterates that life has been worth living; it has been a good life, a happy life, and by all definitions that society uses to judge individuals, Frank has had a successful life.

Frank's experiences are fairly typical of the World War II veteran with a service-connected disability. Their acute SCI management was fairly primitive because of battlefield conditions initially and the general lack of knowledge about long-term SCI management. Thus, this group essentially taught the medical profession about living with a disability and provided the stimulus for the development of the specialty of rehabilitation medicine.

The government benefits provided to service-connected disabled veterans were prompted by gratitude and were an effort to compensate them for a loss incurred while defending our country. Many of the group have chosen to join the work force, some have not. But the government sponsorship provided and continues to provide a level of financial security that gives them complete freedom, within the limits of their disability, to make decisions about how they will live their lives.

CLIFFORD
The Self-Made Man

In November 1936, Clifford, aged 22, was a senior in college when he and a group of friends had an automobile accident in the rural Midwest. Cliff was the only passenger seriously hurt, and he assures you that if he had not acquired his T12-L1 complete spinal injury then, he certainly would have in the process of being extricated from the car, transferred to the local hospital, and sent by train (baggage car) to the big city hospital 60 miles away. Furthermore, the x-ray technicians were determined to get a full visualization of his spine and so they moved him every which way in order to get the proper pictures. The big-city physicians knew what spinal injury was, of course, and thus made no promises about life expectancy. They recommended a laminectomy to release pressure on a badly swollen spinal cord and gave him one chance in a thousand of surviving the surgery. He had zero chances without it. Given those odds, Cliff decided to go for the surgery and awoke post-op to find himself in a full body cast from armpits to knees. The body cast was undisturbed while he lay on his back in the hospital and, not surprisingly, after five weeks he had pressure sores on each hip, the sacral area, and his heels. They sent him home, though, to the family farm, and his mother applied hot soaks and ointments to the pressure sores and his father boiled a rubber catheter three times a day to extract urine from his bladder. His urine was badly infected and to this day he still remembers the horrible smell. But since there were no antibiotics in those days, they flushed the bladder with some purple liquid (perhaps gentian violet) and eventually the bladder infection disappeared. After his pressure sores healed, his father would carry him downstairs to a big cane-backed wheelchair with large wheels in front. In this he could maneuver from the living room to the front porch and watch the world go by. Cliff was told that he would live no more than three years.

Sitting around and doing nothing had never been his lifestyle, so a year and a half after his injury he decided that he would like to walk. The local blacksmith was consulted and eventually he had some braces that covered his legs and went halfway up his body. After several months of teaching himself to ambulate, Cliff went back to the blacksmith, this time to devise hand controls for his stick-shift car. He says that he sure was busy with the steering, clutching, shifting, accelerating, and braking, but he was able to get around on his own and be free again for the first time in two years. In 1938, Cliff's father died, which left him and his mother alone with no income and thus they lost the farm. However, Cliff persuaded the local gentry to appoint him to his father's unexpired term as County Commissioner, which paid $42 a month. Thus, with this as their only income, Cliff and his mother moved into town and he spent many long hours trying to figure out what he could do with his life. Since he knew agriculture, he started to invest part of the $42 into cattle and pigs and soon he was making some decent money. In fact, he was able to buy one of the first automobiles equipped with automatic transmission, a big black Oldmobile, just four days before the start of World War II when auto manufacturing was diverted into the war effort. Later he was elected County Commissioner in his own right for another four-year term and expanded his investments into ranching. Soon he was a landowner, farmer, and rancher and able to hire the help he needed to run the ranch.

Over the years, Cliff never had any rehabilitation but learned how to manage the residuals of his spinal injury through trial and error. He trained his bladder and bowel to empty on schedule and wore pads inside of rubber pants in case of accidents. He continued to walk with braces and crutches and never used a wheelchair.

By 1944, Cliff decided that he would like to become a lawyer. At the time of his injury, he had been studying pre-med but now realized that a profession with more sitting and desk work would be better. Therefore, he went to see the dean of the local law school. The dean remarked that the lack of a bachelor's degree would be a problem because you could not get a law degree without an undergraduate degree. Yet, you did not need a law degree to practice law. You just needed to pass the bar exam. So theoretically Cliff could take the law classes and then pass the bar. "Great idea," said Cliff. "Unfortunately, I can't let you do that," said the dean, "because the rules state that you have to have a bachelor's degree for admission into law school." After dwelling on this for a while and discarding the idea of returning to the state university to finish his undergraduate work (the school was spread out over a large area with many multistory buildings), Cliff petitioned the State Supreme Court to waive the rule and allow him to take classes in the law school. The court did waive the rule, and Cliff completed three years of law courses in one year and nine months.

The cattle and ranching business continued to be successful, which allowed him to support his mother and put himself through school. In addition to working and studying, he found time to sing in several church choirs (his splendid tenor voice was quite in demand) and to date Paula, a law school classmate, whom he married three days after they both passed the state bar exam. Interestingly, her family had no objections to her marriage to a person with a physical disability, nor did his. Perhaps being a civilian who was already actively participating in life created a different image in contrast to all of the publicity surrounding our disabled war veterans who were still hospitalized and expected to die within a few years. For Cliff, marriage occurred nine years after his injury at a time when he had already established himself as a rancher, businessman, politician, and lawyer. One also wonders if walking rather than using a wheelchair defused many of the negative stereotypes associated with disability. Yet, the most likely explanation is unrelated to equipment. Cliff does not think of himself as disabled and, of course, this is a key factor in the successful "adjustment" to all disability.

In September 1946, Clifford and Paula moved back to his hometown and opened a joint law office, but Cliff continued to be involved in ranching throughout his life and had other business interests. At various times he was involved in the funeral business, owned a motel, owned a car dealership, in addition to being actively involved in local and state politics, their joint law practice, and the organization of a regional telephone company. Finally, by the late 1970s, Clifford and Paula had a net worth of over $3 million.

The adoption of children was a roadblock for Clifford and Paula also. There was only one adoption agency in the area and it, too, had rules against placing children in a home in which a parent had a physical disability. They did get involved in the black market in babies but finally the local agency gave in because

Paula had a friend on the board of directors who intervened on their behalf. Thus, two sons joined the family in the late 1950s.

Clifford's story of living with his spinal cord injury is particularly remarkable because he never knew that there was anything that he could not do. He walked throughout most of the years from the onset of his paralysis, and he did not use a wheelchair until 1973 when his hip joints had totally deteriorated from osteoarthritis and no one could figure out how to make an artificial hip function properly without substantial muscle mass to hold it in place. In addition, his wrists were beginning to hurt quite badly from those many years of using crutches, but even so, he resents the wheelchair as a hindrance and a symbol of "giving in" to the disability, something he would never do. At the same time, it must be emphasized that the wheelchair is a liberating device because it adds function that would not be possible with major impairment in the lower extremities. While Cliff understands this, the use of more adaptive equipment is typically postponed until absolutely necessary by most of our older citizens with disabilities.

Cliff's medical history is an extraordinary example of mind over matter, the will to live, and the positive power of emotions on body functions. In total, he has had 30–40 major operations (he has lost count) and has been vulnerable to infections all of his spinal injury life. However, he has never allowed his physical function to interfere with what he wanted to do.

Innumerable bladder infections finally culminated in surgery to insert an artificial sphincter in 1977, which has been replaced numerous times because of malfunction. He had a rectal fistula and surgery for this problem several times in the early 1950s, a prolapsed rectum in 1971, which prolapsed again in 1974, resulting in a colostomy complicated by peritonitis. In 1960 and 1964, a testicle was removed because of chronic infection and because it seemed to be transmitting other infections. In 1973, the head of a femur was removed; in 1974, his gallbladder was removed; and since 1977, he has been on antibiotics to prevent bladder infections. Pressure sores have not been a major problem but there have been a few. His feet would swell and the rubbing of his braces against his ankles often aggravated a sore, but these tended to heal readily. Only recently has he started using a cushion in his wheelchair (1984), and, because of shoulder discomfort, he is now using a sliding board for transfers. Cliff has never been inside of a rehabilitation center, expects to have to instruct all physicians about how he needs to be treated for his spinal injury, and believes that most professionals are too paternalistic toward disabled people and take away the necessity of learning to take care of themselves. Without a doubt, he believes in keeping going at all costs and never slows down enough to dwell on difficulties. Life has been hard, physically hard, but life has been good and by all standards by which we judge each other, Clifford has had a successful life.

The recent years have involved some bad luck that has brought financial insecurity for the first time since the depression of the 1930s. The man who operated the car dealership for him mismanaged the company and diverted funds for his own use. Thus, Clifford and Paula had to cover a tremendous financial loss in the early 1980s at a time when their cattle caught brucellosis and could not be sold. The bank foreclosed, they sold what they could and moved south to "retire." Their income derives from Social Security and his salary as an employee of a loan brokerage business. His medical expenses amount to over $200 a month, some of which is covered by Medicare. However, given his medical history, they face considerable monthly expense. Blue Cross of their home state cancelled their policy and new medical insurance has proven to be difficult to obtain and costly when obtainable. Paula has been an income tax specialist in the past and plans to take a refresher course on recent tax law in order to add to their income and prepare for those times when Cliff cannot work because of medical problems. Neither Paula nor Clifford dwell on this turn of events but rather continue to be the resourceful, proud, and dynamic people they have always been. While they had not expected to face financial insecurity again, especially at a time when their energy is flagging, they tend to view their glass as half full rather than half empty. This is most certainly why Clifford, with the support of his family, has been able to make medical history. It is probable that no one else has survived and lived as fully with so many medical problems after spinal injury as Cliff has. For 50 years, he has defied the odds and would not permit his body to quit. He is a most remarkable man.

Clifford is the epitome of the self-made man, whether disabled or "nondisabled." He had no rehabilitation and no disabled role models to help and advise him. Thus, rather than vegetate, he move forcefully ahead into all avenues of life. In many ways he has never known how to be "disabled."

Clifford has never received any monies that were not earned through his own efforts; through great intelligence, drive, and good business sense, he has managed a degree of independence not often achieved by individuals with disabilities without some financial assistance (or by people without disabilities). But within either a disabled or "nondisabled" group, such dynamic self-made men account for a small percentage of us, and few can accomplish what he has without some help. He had achieved a level of financial security that gave him freedom to live his life the way he wanted. However, now he is very vulnerable financially as he faces declining energy and more disability with age.

SALLY
The Disabled Woman—A Dual-Minority Status

Sally, a 55-year-old woman with three grown children, has lived with her spinal cord injury for 49 years. Actually, she is not certain as to how she acquired the injury but believes that it resulted from being hit in the neck with a baseball bat at age six. She never even told her parents about it. Her neck was sore for a while, but only months later did she begin to have trouble walking. After falling down repeatedly, she was hospitalized and the medical staff pondered what could possibly be the problem. Perhaps is was curvature of the spine or even polio, the physicians thought, but they were not certain what was wrong. Until age eight, she was in and out of the hospital, mostly in, and usually in traction. Soon she could not walk at all. During this time her mother had a "nervous breakdown" and was sent to the state mental institution for several years. Her father took care of her and her two older sisters as best he could until her mother resumed some family roles when Sally was a teenager. Unfortunately, although the family was caring, she was trapped at home without any of the usual activities that young people normally experience and thus was virtually a prisoner of her disability.

Sally never had any real rehabilitation; in fact, she is not certain of the exact level of her spinal cord injury. My assessment is C8-T1 (eighth cervical vertebra and first thoracic), since she has almost normal hand function but not full dexterity. After getting out of the hospital at age eight, Sally attended regular school, but her repeated bladder accidents were terribly embarrassing and the children made fun of her. It was a horrible time in her life. Several years later she was transferred to a school for children with orthopedic disabilities. Luckily the teachers and staff knew about physical disability problems, and they began to teach her some techniques of self-care and mobility, the only instruction in these matters that she ever received.

After graduation from high school in the early 1950s, she obtained a job as an office clerk for two and a half years, which provided her first taste of independence and freedom. For transportation she relied on a taxi each way, which absorbed half of her salary, but it was worth it to be out of the house and active. The office closed, unfortunately, but after much searching she was hired as a switchboard operator.

After graduation, Sally finally had the chance to have a social life but this was cut short when she got pregnant in 1953. She was naive and inexperienced in matters of dating and had never received any sex education. Why would a disabled woman need to know about such matters? Besides, no man would be interested in a woman with a disability. These were the attitudes prevalent then and, to some degree, today also. Her pregnancy, of course, was "shameful" (yet, at the same time, an entrée into "normalcy"), so she moved out of town to live with one of her sisters until her son, Harold, was born. Eventually returning to her parents' home, she received Aid to Dependent Children (ADC) of $50 a month and did clerical work part-time in the house. Again she found herself trapped.

When Harold was six, Sally married Alex after dating him for a year. Working in the local factory, he made enough money for them to have a reasonably good life, but unfortunately he had a drinking problem which got worse each year. In 1960, Frank was born, and Mary arrived in 1964. By the late 1960s, the marriage had become a nightmare and there was no way that she could physically escape the stress other than to go into the bedroom and shut the door when he began yelling. Since she couldn't drive, she was literally dependent on her husband, who became more dysfunctional over time. Finally he hit her.

That was the last straw, so to speak, and she immediately filed a complaint with the police, which resulted in a one-year probation for him. In that regard, he learned a lesson and never hit her again even though he continually threatened her physically and psychologically. Four times she kicked him out of the house; he would repent, shape up for a while, and then the old pattern would start again. Finally, in 1971, she filed for a legal separation and he moved out. Alex paid child support for one year and then the payments stopped. ADC plus Social Security Disability Insurance (SSDI) were her only sources of support.

As she separated from Alex, Sally realized that she could count on no one but herself. Her father finally taught her to drive, and she bought a car with money that she had earned from clerical work. In 1971, she found a little house and bought it with an FHA loan on which she still makes payments. In order to survive, in order to have enough money to live on, she worked part-time doing clerical work even though the RULES of our social welfare programs stipulate that income of over $400 a month results in loss of Medicaid and Social Security benefits. She feels terrible that she is forced to cheat in order to have enough money to live on, since it is certainly impossible on her SSDI allotment of $399 and her Supplemental Security Income (SSI) of $42 a month to cover expenses. One son is at home and contributes money from his salary, the other is married and lives in another city, and Mary is away at college, earning her education through her own efforts.

Sally represents the majority of persons with physical disability in the United States who are faced with a patchwork quilt of social legislation, the benefits and rules for qualification of each being different. These programs are not co-ordinated with each other to meet the needs of persons with disabilities; in fact, sometimes eligibility for one precludes eligibility for another despite the fact that both programs may be necessary for survival. It is difficult to get information as to what programs are available and often the exclusionary rules are positively draconian—not by deliberate intent of policymakers but from fragmentation of coverage and lack of understanding as to what living with a disability entails. These rules frequently penalize efforts to be independent and self-sufficient and convey the message, "If you are poor, you deserve it." Most people with physical disabilities are poor (because it costs more to live with a disability) and therefore need to be extremely resourceful in order to survive. This resourcefulness includes frugality, creativity, and the ability to work the system: learning the rules and learning how to bend the rules. We must realize that bending the rules and playing the game with taxpayers' dollars is often considered part of the American free enterprise system, and that physically disabled people may occasionally do this in order to have the bare minimum of food and shelter; the media report every day that many top-level individuals and corporations do the very same thing.

Throughout her life with spinal injury, Sally has had to tolerate and ignore a "pins and needles" pain in her spine that is always there. In 1971, she began using a catheter so that she would not have to transfer to the toilet as frequently. Switching to an electric wheelchair eased the shoulder and arm pain from years of transfers but this necessitated the purchase of a van with hydraulic lifts. Recently, osteoporosis has been an increasing problem, and, thus, she has broken her leg several times by not being as careful as she should about placement of her feet. Edema (swelling) in the lower extremities occurs frequently, which makes it difficult to find shoes that do not cause pressure sores. Bladder infections seem to be occurring more frequently, every several months, but the big worry is the headache and hypertension associated with autonomic dysreflexia (sudden rise in the blood pressure in those with spinal injury at T6 and above). Sometimes any movement will trigger it; sometimes her bowel program brings on an attack; and when the dysreflexia comes, it may last for days. The local physicians know nothing about such problems and she has had trouble convincing the local emergency room (ER) that this is a life-threatening crisis. After repeated visits to the same ER, some of the personnel have a general idea of how to help her. But no one is interested in finding the cause of these repeated episodes or in helping her to prevent them from occurring. "You can expect to have such problems as you get older so you are going to have to learn to live with these things," the physicians tell her. At this point in the interview, weeping, she describes how abandoned she feels by the medical community. The new Medicare and Medicaid rulings state that, if one is admitted to the hospital without a specific diagnosis, payment may not be approved and then she would be responsible for the bill. Thus, the physicians are reluctant to admit her when she is having a major episode of autonomic dysreflexia, since they do not understand the nature of the problem. It is interesting to note that Sally resides, not in the boondocks, but in a major American city with a reputable medical school and two major rehabilitation centers, one of which is directed by a nationally known physiatrist. When asked if she had contacted school X, rehabilitation centers A & B, and Dr. Z, she replied that they were only interested in newly spinal-injured persons, and they seemed to lose interest in you once you were out of the hospital. Currently, with stipends supplemented by her own earnings, she is just getting by financially, and she has no extra money to save for the future as her function declines. She has never had a vacation and still makes payments on her little house, which is now in an unsafe part of town. Unfortunately, she cannot afford to move. Occasionally, Sally finds herself worrying about the future and what will happen when she can no longer be independent. The local independent living center has a program to train personal care attendants and maintain a registry of available personnel, but some of her friends have had horrible experiences with psychologically unsuitable aides who try to transform them into virtual prisoners in their own home. Unfortunately, when one needs physical help in order to survive, one often is forced to tolerate a terrible situation because of the apparent lack of alternatives. It is important to note that independent living centers (ILC) have filled a great void in the service network for people with disabilities; however, they vary in the effectiveness of their component programs.

Despite all of this, Sally asserts that she has had a happy life and that she has been happiest since Alex moved out and she was able to acquire her own home and car. Finally, she had gained control over her own life and did not have to accommodate to the wishes of parents or husband. After 49 years with spinal cord injury, she has had only 15 years of independence and it has been wonderful. However, as she grows older, she fears that she will again lose her precious ability to govern her own life. Motherhood has been a great pleasure but she regrets that she missed all of the PTA meetings, school plays, or parent-teacher conferences because the schools were inaccessible. Early in her marriage when the stress became extreme, she joined the Catholic Church and has found great comfort in her religious beliefs. "If I did not know and believe that there was life after death, I would not have gotten to this point. There has to be more to look forward to than this."

Currently, she tries to take each day at a time and makes an effort not to think of the future or else she will get depressed. Yet, Sally is an extremely resourceful, charming, and creative person who has exhibited great strength and determination in living with her spinal injury. "You have got to take care of yourself," she says. "You cannot expect anyone to do it for you. But if only there were a reliable system of services to help me to stay in my own home as I get older. I don't want to go to a nursing home."

Sally also had no rehabilitation, but with a much more severe physical disability and with the role of woman, she was faced with a dual minority status, and both have penalized her attempts to exert full control over her life. [The topic of the double disability of the physically impaired woman is eloquently addressed by Deegan and Brooks (1985).] Despite being a sheltered daughter and abused wife, she has overcome these delimiting environmental circumstances to challenge her physical disability through hard work and resourcefulness. As a woman and as a disabled woman from a low-income family, she had no opportunity to acquire advanced education in order to obtain a high-salaried job, even though she is extremely bright. Thus, she has had to settle for survival without the hope of achieving much more, but at least it has been done on her own terms for the last 15 years. In one sense, freedom cannot be purchased because it is a state of mind. However, for those with physical disabilities who thereby have lost a variety of options, freedom is often synonymous with having a significant amount of income.

JACK
The Nonservice-Connected Disabled Veteran

Jack has lived with his spinal injury (T10) for 31 years since he fell off a roof while working as a carpenter. He was 29, married with two children under two years of age, and just starting to establish himself in life. Because he was self-employed at the time, he did not qualify for Worker's Compensation, and, thus, his accident became not only a personal but a financial disaster. During his one and a half years of hospitalization, his wife and children counted on ADC for their income, supplemented by what little she could earn as a temporary secretarial helper. As Jack recalls, ADC in 1956 had particularly restrictive regulations designed to ensure that only the most destitute people received help. And, indeed, his family became destitute. They were not allowed to own a car or have a telephone, so Jack's father purchased the car from them and let them "borrow" it, and his brother paid for the telephone. In order to work, his wife had to pay for a babysitter, so it was close to a "no win" game. Fortunately, they received $50 a month by mail from an anonymous donor for a year, and they still wonder who sent it. That $50 made the difference between eating and not eating on many occasions, even though it was usually only beans or macaroni and cheese for dinner.

Because he had been in the military earlier, he was eligible for free care at the VA hospital as a nonservice-connected disabled veteran. In the 10 years since World War II, acute treatment was vastly more enlightened so that Jack received physical and occupational therapy to teach him to be independent. Nevertheless, his hospitalization lasted 18 months, whereas today the initial hospitalization for a new paraplegic in the civilian sector averages approximately 90 days.

After discharge from the hospital, Jack obtained a full-time job in a paper partition factory, bought a car with automatic transmission, and designed and constructed the hand controls himself in order to save money. He and his wife believed that a mother should stay at home with the children; thus, their only income was from his salary. Unfortunately, when he developed a medical problem that kept him from work, the factory's disability income insurance policy did not cover him, and, thus, the family had no money during these times. The ruling stated that if he could work at the factory, he was by definition not disabled. Furthermore, any medical problems secondary to his spinal cord injury were not considered to be evidence of disability, and so he did not qualify for disability income.

Jack hated being paralyzed and viewed his accident as a terrrible hardship for his family. Now the "Catch-22" situation of the disability income insurance was the last straw, so to speak, and he attempted suicide, not once but twice, both exceedingly serious attempts. However when he realized how much his wife loved him and that his suicide attempts were only adding to her burden, he decided to make the best of his situation. After 10 years of full-time work at the factory, it became apparent that Jack and his family would be slightly better off financially by his not working! His job paid $4.50 and hour or $180 a week, on which he had to pay taxes and buy insurance, and his income stopped when he was away from work with medical problems. Consequently, in 1967 he quit work and accepted a VA nonservice-connected disability pension, plus aid and attendant's allowance, and his wife went to work in the local school lunch program. Currently, he receives approximately $800 a month (VA plus SSI) plus his wife's salary nine months of the year. His medical care is free at the local VA, but service-connected veterans receive top priority. As a nonservice-connected veteran, he may have to wait for admission until a bed becomes available. Upon his death, his wife will receive no money from the VA and her only income will be from her Social Security and a small pension from the school. They own their own home, which is mortgage free, and have $10,000 insurance. However, in the 31 years since his accident, they have never been able to afford to go away on vacation. They have had only enough money to live on.

Since leaving the job, life has not been any easier for Jack because time hangs heavily on his hands. "I'm not very intelligent," Jack says in a matter-of-fact manner. "I've never enjoyed reading or intellectual activities." Before the accident he used to be very active and independent, but he was always physically oriented, not intellectually oriented. He feels useless around the house as he watches his wife struggle and work hard. He is, however, mechanically inclined, and for the last eight years he has been volunteering many hours a week at the VA occupational therapy department designing and making adaptive equipment for patients.

According to Jack, aging has not been a major problem for him. He is 61 now but has lived with the spinal injury 10 years less than the World War II fellows who are the same age. Also, his acute SCI treatment was certainly better. He gets shoulder and arm tenderness occasionally, and, from the moment of injury, he has had a burning pain in his back. A vesicostomy and colostomy were performed years ago, and there have been no pressure sore problems since the early years. Thus, from his point of view, except for hypertension for the last five years, his physical function is not very different than it has been.

Life has not been easy for Jack and his wife, and so I asked him what would have made his life better. At the top of his list was a change in disability income regulations that would permit a person to work and have a reasonable income. Not working has been psychologically devastating to this man and has been more "disabling" than his spinal cord injury. "Yes but," one might say, "if he really had the right stuff, he would have overcome his predicament." Yet, this is only a variation on the self-fulfilling prophecy, "If you are poor, you deserve it." In his own way, Jack has shown as much strength as Frank, Clifford, and Sally, but he, perhaps, had fewer resources to fall back on because he does not have superior intelligence. Furthermore, he grew up with the idea of being a skilled laborer and had no concept of another way of life. He expected to work; he believed that a man should support his wife, and this is what he wanted to do. But living with a disability is expensive and it requires a significantly greater income just to survive than for nondisabled people. The average person with a disability who does not qualify for a high-paying job often finds that the income earned barely covers living expenses. Because one is employed, one may not qualify for Medicaid, and, therefore, one cannot afford the medical expenses secondary to life with a disability. At least Jack qualified for free care at the VA because of his veteran status, but nonveterans have two routes: private medical insurance (which often excludes conditions associated with preexisting disability) or Medicaid. If you earn more than "$X" per month, you lose eligibility for Medicaid (rules vary by state of residence), and, for this reason, many persons with disabilities find that they cannot afford to work because of the cost of medical care, another "Catch 22."

Jack's life had also been compromised by inaccessible housing. There are many areas of his own home that are inaccessible to him because they could not afford to make the necessary modifications or to buy a more properly designed house. The major obstacles are steps, narrow doorways, narrow hallways, and inaccessible bathrooms. The family has little money for recreation but finds that the wheelchair-accessible seats at local arenas and theatres are in the top price category. This, frankly, is quite cruel, since, as a group, people with disabilities have less money available than "nondisabled" folks.

Without a doubt, Jack's wife has been a major supportive factor in his life, but not working has been a devastating experience for him. Life with a physical disability has been bad enough, but Jack's self-image as a man has been challenged by the fact that he could not earn enough to support his family. He has tolerated a difficult situation for many years, but, when he goes to bed at night, he almost wishes he wouldn't wake up. "Thirty-one years is enough," Jack says.

For Jack, the physical disability has deprived him of many options that were essential to his well-being: working independently and supporting his family on his income alone. In addition to the penalty of being disabled, he was also penalized financially by a variety of regulations that kept lowering his income when he worked outside of the home. Unfortunately, he did not have the intellectual abilities to gain an advanced degree or become an entrepreneurial businessman like Clifford, and thus, like Sally, he has had to settle for mere survival. However, unlike Sally, it has not been on his own terms. His has been a life of imprisonment by his disability, by his definition of manhood and by the social legislation of the last three decades.

PAUL

A Man Covered by Worker's Compensation

Paul's story is quite different from our previous ones in that he has lived with his spinal cord injury only 14 years; only 14 years, but these were supposed to be the golden years. Paul is now 74 years old and acquired a C5-6 quadriplegia in an auto accident while on a business trip. Betty, his wife, recalls the phone call from the hospital advising her not to come because he was paralyzed from the neck down and not expected to live. Needless to say, she hopped the first plane available and stayed at his side for the next several months. After the acute injury was stabilized, he had to choose a rehabilitation center, the very good one in his hometown or an even better one many miles away. He chose to return to his hometown, and in his case, this turned out to be a critically important decision. Paul spent many hours lying on a bed believing that life was over and wondering what he could possibly "do" for the rest of his life. Now even his most basic activities of feeding, grooming, bathing, and dressing were not under his control, and he would need attendant care for the rest of his life.

Paul had been managing editor of a major newspaper but now could not type or do any of the things he believed were necessary for the job. However, his hospital roommate, a university professor with a recent spinal injury, did not have such doubts about what he would do and continued to monitor graduate students' progress and hold seminars at his bedside. Paul, as he recalls, caught the habit and soon was conferring with reporters, junior editors, and his secretary about daily newspaper activities. With encouragement from his colleagues, Paul started to believe that he could "do" something, in fact, he could do what he had always loved: journalism. But the logistics of adapting the telephone, typewritter, office, and daily work schedule to the demands of his quadriplegia seemed overwhelming at times, and seemingly minor impediments became major obstacles to function. However, when his morale was at its lowest, he saw a quadriplegic man in a business suit and vest, obviously actively involved in professional activities, which reminded him that others had overcome similar obstacles. (This is a perfect example of the importance of role models during critical periods in disabled people's lives.) Consequently, nine months after the accident, he returned to work and maintained an almost perfect work record until he retired at age 65.

Paul willingly states that he could not have returned to work without the support of his wife and without the financial support provided by Worker's Compensation. All medical expenses associated with the spinal injury, medications, and attendant care are covered for the rest of his life. Most particularly he could not have returned to work without the services of an attendant and access to his own transportation.

After retirement, Paul and Betty moved south, which brought a whole new set of adjustments. Finding and keeping good attendants is a constant issue in their lives, since Paul needs help with the most basic activities of daily living. Furthermore, he is a big man, 6'4", and therefore, a lot to handle. Consequently, an attendent comes in seven days a week for four hours in the morning, and Betty helps him during the remainder of the day and evening. This naturally constricts Betty's freedom even though she will go out without him for tennis, shopping, or an occasional lunch. She knows that she needs time for herself and Paul insists that he does not need her there all the time, but she worries about him while she is out. So she does not go out a great deal. Betty is nearing 70 years old and is in comparatively good health, but aches and pains are becoming a part of her life too. Both enjoy the south but find the heat in the summer to be a major limitation on the scope of their activities. Since Paul has an impaired temperature regulation system (which occurs in SCI above T4-6), he cannot be in extremes of heat or cold for very long. Unfortunately, the air conditioning system in their van does not provide rapid enough response and low enough temperatures to ensure Paul's safety. Otherwise they would love to travel in the summer, but, of course, it is a problem to find attendant care in any vacation location or even when visiting relatives. Thus, they tend to stay in town and spend most of their time inside their own home during a large part of the summer season.

Paul had been a workaholic prior to retirement, and, therefore, not being at work presented a new challenge of what he would "do." (For men in our society, "doing" has been closely associated with working.) So he proceeded to learn to like a whole new set of activities: watching TV sports events and listening to classical music, for example. He had always been an avid reader, but now holding the book and page turning require proper positioning and is not as spontaneous an activity for quadriplegics as for others.

Paul reports few problems associated with aging that seem to be related to the disability itself. His bowels are slowing down as often happens in later years, but the constellation of problems reported by those who have lived a longer period with the disability does not seem to bother him at this time. Admittedly, however, Paul is less capable of independent physical acitivity than many and, thus, does not have the opportunity to put excessive stress on muscles and joints.

Paul and Betty have no financial worries currently, since they had invested wisely and saved for retirement. However, his medical expenses amount to almost $15,000 a year now, in addition to which they pay $13,200 a year for personal care attendants. Without Worker's Compensation, all of their wise planning for the future would be obliterated by the magnitude of such additional yearly expenses required for him to survive with his quadriplegia.

These people are dynamic, resourceful, and stoic. They maintain a good outlook on life and a good sense of humor despite the difficulties of the last 14 years. However, when I commented that no one envisions retirement under quite the circumstances that they now face, Betty, a grandmotherly woman who could fit easily into a Norman Rockwell painting, said, "As far as we're concerned, you can screw the golden years."

Paul certainly has been penalized by his disability but also receives money as partial compensation for his losses acquired as a working man. Without this financial compensation, he would not be able to live independently with his wife in their own home because of his age, his size, and the severity of his disability. Long ago their well-laid financial plans for retirement would have been demolished by the magnitude of the yearly expenses associated with his disability. He is an intelligent, resourceful, and hard-working man, but these personal assets would not be enough to overcome the magnitude of the expense of his physical disability. Thus, Paul is "lucky"—lucky that, if he had to acquire a physical disability, it happened while he was at work.

DAVE
The Civilian with Few Environmental Resources

At age 17, Dave was maneuvering his motorcycle down a dark highway when a car inexplicably backed up across the road, blocking his path. The accident resulted in a C7-T1 quadriplegia for Dave and a $15 fine for the driver. This was 1949 in the rural western part of the United States. The local general hospital to which Dave was admitted knew nothing about spinal cord injury, and, as a result, he acquired pressure sores on his buttocks within a day or two. Six weeks later, they transferred him to a big city hospital for evaluation of his neurological status only. Luckily, these physicians knew more about SCI and recommended surgery to repair the pressure sores. This took six months and two operations. However, even in this comparatively enlightened establishment, there was no rehabilitation and he received therapy only for range of motion of his extremities by a physical therapist. Despite his objections, Dave was returned to his local hospital, and, as he feared, the professional staff had learned little about SCI in his absence. For example, spasticity had started in his lower extremities; their solution was stretching, so he was placed in long leg braces for two years. It did not work; he still had spasticity, which was later relieved through surgery. Living in a 50-bed ward was a terrible experience; consequently, Dave asked to go home. The physicians were certain that this would not work out, and Dave too had his concerns about this but for different reasons. He had left home originally because he and his stepfather did not get along; however, anything was better than the hospital. Needless to say, Dave's stepfather was decidedly unenthusiastic about his wife's son coming back into the house so the man built a very small "lean-to" shed on the outside of the farmhouse as a residence for his stepson. Thus it was in this shed that Dave lived for the next four years.

Meanwhile, Dave's mother tried to pursue legal remedies regarding the accident. Their attorney, however, advised her to settle for $4,000, even though the driver was using a company car and personally had a $100,000 liability insurance policy. The attorney took $1,000 for his "services," and the remainder was put in trust for Dave until he reached 21. Until that age, he received $65 a month from the trust fund.

During the next several years, Dave lay in bed in his shed trying to figure out what he could do to gain control over his life again. When he reached 21 and gained access to his trust fund, he gave the money to his stepfather to build a bedroom onto the house so that he could finally come indoors. After buying a hospital bed and a wheelchair, Dave had $300 left, which he used to start a mail order postage stamp business. The Department of Vocational Rehabilitation (DVR) assisted by giving him a used electric typewriter and a thermofax copier to get started. From this base, Dave became an entrepreneur, purchasing stamps from the post office and collectors, advertising his acquisitions, and selling the stamps by mail to people around the country. Gradually, the business grew to the point that he was making $100 a month, but, no matter what he did, he could not earn more without additional capital to expand the business. Lack of transporation was a further hindrance. By 1960, he realized that he was at a dead end, so he decided to go to college. However, when he applied to DVR for financial assistance, they refused, stating that his case was closed because he already had been "rehabilitated."

Dave was determined to get out of his stepfather's house, where he was virtually a prisoner in his own room. It was a risky step but he phased out his business and sold two-thirds of the inventory in order to obtain money to purchase a mobile home. Apartment living would be too expensive in the long run, he calculated. For $800 he bought an 8' × 27' unit, which he was able to sell for $600 18 months later in order to buy a larger one already made accessible for wheelchair living. The mobile home space cost $30 a month; he had no transportation; he lived on Aid to the Totally Disabled (ATD); and in 1964, 15 years after his accident, he enrolled at the state college, despite DVR's refusal to sponsor him. Biology was his first love, but psychology seemed more practical for someone in a wheelchair so that became his major. Unfortunately, most of the psych courses were scheduled in rooms on the second floor and there were no elevators. So Dave discussed this with the dean of the school who promised to change the class location, but the course instructor objected. The dean was chagrined and claimed helplessness to remedy the situation. As a result of this experience, Dave learned to approach the instructor himself whenever a class was inaccessible and none ever refused to change the room assignment. "You can't count on others to get the job done for you. You are better off by doing it yourself," Dave says.

During college, Dave survived on ATD, plus whatever he could earn from his remaining stamp business. Lacking transportation, he had to hire someone to drive him to school and back so he scheduled all his classes to occur on Tuesdays and Thursdays in order to save money. Since there were no disabled student services, Dave learned to fend for himself, to read regulations and eligibility requirements very carefully, and to use face-to-face contact to get what he needed. Thus, he learned to be an advocate, initially for himself and later for others.

In the process of organizing a local chapter of the National Paraplegia Foundation Dave met many key people in the state, one of whom promised to intervene for him with DVR for financial aid with his college expenses. DVR did agree to help him out, but only with registration fees, not with books. Eventually, however, because much of the college was inaccessible to him, Dave decided to move to a larger city within the state that had a more accessible state college campus and more opportunities for disabled people within the city itself. DVR agreed to the move; he bought a car for $50, paid someone to move his mobile home, and waited for DVR to contact him about resuming school.

Meanwhile, Dave decided to have his bladder status monitored at the local rehabilitation center. However, the rules stated that a person could be treated in the outpatient department only if they had been seen as in inpatient previously. Consequently, he got himself admitted as an inpatient but then had a difficult time convincing the staff that he had only wanted admission in order to be discharged. Besides, he had a stamp business to run with schedules and deadlines to be met and he really had to get back to school. Nevertheless, the team sprang into action and planned all sorts of evaluations and training on how to do his self-care differently. He protested and remained adamant that he knew what he was doing and did not want to change his methods. Finally, after a two-week stand-off, they discharged him to his desired status of "outpatient." Actually, Dave believes that they were secretly relieved to get rid of him, especially when they discovered that he was counseling newly injured SCI on how to take charge of their own lives and make their own decisions.

Since he still had not heard from DVR, he contacted them only to find out that they had closed his case, not transferred it. After re-applying for assistance from DVR, he decided not to wait for their decision and enrolled in college immediately and applied for financial assistance from the college. They did not offer financial aid; however, they did offer him a job! So Dave went to school full-time, worked in the college placement office, worked on his stamp business, and got $150 a month from ATD. This provided just enough income to survive.

In 1971, Dave graduated with a B.S. in psychology but discovered that there were few jobs available that did not require more advanced degrees. As a result, he enrolled in graduate school and volunteered at the state college as a disabled student services counselor, essentially developing a program for them. This experience turned out to be very helpful because he was offered a job in a similar program at a nearby community college two years later. Finally, he was able to phase out his stamp business entirely, but as a person with quadriplegia living alone he still could not survive on just his salary. He needed state assistance. In the mid 1970s, Dave became very active in the disability rights movement, took courses in graduate school, taught a class on rights and resources for the disabled at the state college (which became a model for such courses nationally), served on the board of directors of several disability organizations, was elected a state delegate to the White House Conference on Handicapped Individuals, lobbied in Washington, D.C., for more enlightened social legislation regarding the disabled, and worked three-quarter time at his job. He had a fully independent life: living alone in his own mobile home, driving his own car, hiring the attendant care and homemaking services that he needed. But by 1978, this pace started to exact its toll. Dave noticed increasing fatigue, lowered resistance to infections, along with a marked aggravation of his allergies. Today, he believes that perhaps he took on too much in the 1970s; yet, he cannot be certain that his present decline in function would not have happened even if he had been less active.

Dave worries about the future, perhaps too much, and devotes considerable mental energy to planning for every possible contingency. It is just such meticulous planning that has allowed him the freedom to leave his parents' home and to be independent. However, at the present, aging and declining energy have introduced even greater uncertainties into his life, something that Dave does not handle well. Thus, currently his biggest challenge is to modulate the very traits that have served him so well in the past.

The daily process of wheeling himself around campus and across many carpeted floors, in addition to transferring in and out of his car, became so exhausting that Dave finally got an electric wheelchair and a van with a hydraulic lift.

Now 54 years old, he has lived with his spinal injury for 37 years, has been meticulous about his self-care, has had few medical problems, but now worries about his loss of energy and the implications of this for independent living. Dave has been so self-sufficient all of his life that he does not know how to rely on anyone else. In fact, most of his personal experience has demonstrated that you can only count on yourself to get things done right. Consequently, the future as a quadriplegic alone is worrisome.

Two years ago, Dave married a woman who had been serving as his personal care attendant. She is a graduate student, highly intelligent, and they got along well together. Getting married always entails a life change, but marriage for the first time at age 52 after a lifetime of total self-reliance is a major adjustment, and Dave is feeling the stress. Having a wife, in one sense, is an attempt to reduce stress associated with being alone and disabled, but having a wife introduces new stresses that he never anticipated. Dave is an orderly and compulsive person who likes to be in control of everything and to plan things down to the last detail. Thus, the whole pattern of living that has worked so successfully for him is challenged by the need to take into account another person's wishes. Furthermore, two cannot live as cheaply as one, Dave has discovered.

His salary brings in $700 a month, after deductions, for 10 months a year. They get an attendant care allowance from the state of $700 a month (if he were not married, it would be $900!), which is taxable also. Consequently, their net income is approximately $1,300 a month. Her graduate program is requiring more and more of her time; thus, they recently hired someone to help Dave when she cannot be there. His mobile home, ideal for one, is too small for two, so he wonders if he should withdraw the money in his retirement pension program at the college to purchase a larger unit. Will the marriage last? It is too soon to tell.

Dave gets depressed these days and agrees that he worries too much, but it is difficult to break a lifetime habit of planning, planning, planning. One of the problems of aging is the decline in energy, which seems to reduce his ability to handle the daily stress of life with a disability. Thus, he gets irritable and depressed more easily these days. Unfortunately, it is not unreasonable to expect that his energy level will decline further, but he has no savings to count on. After a lifetime of resourcefulness and hard work, he was barely able to earn a survival-level income to enable him to be free. Consequently, there was never any extra money to put away for the future, and Dave is a very frugal person.

Today, Dave sometimes wonders if the struggle has been worth it. He is tired and disillusioned. The comradeship and enthusiasm of the disability rights movement of the 1970s has waned, and changes have occurred at a painfully slow pace. Our social legislation has somewhat more enlightened elements than 20 years ago, partly through the efforts of Dave and his colleagues. Yet, you have to study the regulations constantly, keep up with new programs, and always take an assertive stance with the bureaucracies. You have to fight the system, work the system, and bend the rules just to survive. Thus, Dave asks,

"Why did they bother to keep us alive if they are going to make it so difficult for us to live?"

Dave, too, has been penalized both by an extensive disability and by few environmental resources, and therefore has had to settle for mere survival. His high intelligence and determination have helped him to gain his freedom from family, but financial survival has been a constant battle for him. Only his tremendous personal resources, with some governmental help, have allowed him to escape from his parents' home and manage his own life. But the change in his physical condition, the decline in energy, is limiting this freedom, and, consequently, the future is uncertain. He has devoted the major portion of his adult life to educating legislators and policymakers on the reality of life with a disability. But change is slow and now he worries about how long he can afford to remain a free man.

BILL
A Professional Man with the Residuals of Polio

Bill knew what polio was in the early 1950s and he was definitely afraid of catching it. However, when he felt sick with a terrible headache, he blamed it on the flu; he did not think of polio at all. When his back began to hurt badly and his bladder refused to empty, he finally went to a doctor who hospitalized him immediately. Bill remembers walking into the ward and seeing all the iron lungs in rows and wondering, "Why are they putting me in here? I might catch polio from these guys." Even though he caused a stir by walking into the ward (everyone else came in on gurneys), he could not get out of bed by the next morning. Unfortunately, the spinal tap confirmed the diagnosis: poliomyelitis. The paralysis began in his legs and rose to the midthoracic level; his bladder refused to empty without an indwelling catheter; and the sensation in his lower extremities was altered. The latter two symptoms are rarely associated with polio, but there was no question of the diagnosis. Theoretically, we believe that sensation is unimpaired in polio because the disease only hits the motor nerves, but, while he never lost sensation completely, Bill's sensation in the lower half of his body was definitely abnormal. Bill knows what he is talking about; he has since become a physician.

Airplanes were his first love and, until his eyesight required correction by glasses, he had dreamed of becoming a pilot. However, the future had not been a big concern to him and his working-class family did not think of college as an option. But now as a senior in high school, paralyzed from polio, he took life more seriously and wondered if medicine would be available to him as a career. First, however, he had to recover, or so he hoped. Immobilized in bed for the first several months, he had developed a pronounced scoliosis of the spine by the time they allowed him to sit up. Apparently, the muscles on the right side of his body were recovering faster than those on the left, which pulled his spine out of alignment. After five months of hospitalization, he was walking with two long leg braces, crutches, and a corset for his trunk. Luckily, his bladder function returned to normal. Outpatient physical therapy and limited time out of bed prevented him from returning to school that year, but the next year he returned to complete his senior classes. Surgery for scoliosis was scheduled for five days after graduation.

That summer the physicians fused part of his spine from the lower thoracic levels into the upper lumbar region. This improved his function significantly so that he could give up braces and crutches and think about college. Because his family had little money, the high school held a benefit to provide a college scholarship for him, as did the local Kiwanis organization. The staff in the state DVR believed that medicine was an unreasonable goal, however, and suggested that he try bookkeeping or taxi driving rather than college. "Well, I'm going to go to college with or without your help," Bill said, so they agreed to give him a trial. Four years later, he graduated with a bachelor's degree in chemistry and was accepted into medical school, but finances were still a problem. By working as a night watchman during college he had managed to save enough to pay for the first semester in medical school, but he did not know where the money would come from after that. Luckily, the federal student loan program came to his rescue because, without it, becoming a physician would have been an impossibility.

Bill got through the basic science years without trouble, but by his third year in medical school, the clinical years, he noticed increased back pain and fatigue. Nevertheless, he kept pushing himself until he fainted in the operating room during a clinical assignment in surgery. Back home, he went for another operation, this time to extend the fusion higher into the thoracic and lower into the lumbar levels of his spine. Since he was confined to bed in a full-body cast for six months, he lost a year of school but resumed his full schedule the following year. Twelve months later, the pain started again; this was the first in a series of pseudarthroses. The fusion did not hold and either there was a fracture or a nonunion, which resulted in a "false joint," permitting movement where there should be none. The result was terrible pain. After another fusion and another six months in bed, the x-ray films revealed bad news: the fusion did not heal. Harrington rods were still an experimental procedure in parts of the country in 1965, but Bill volunteered for this surgery in the hope that this would solve the problem. So for the fourth time he spent six months in a body cast in bed, but this time it worked.

He graduated in 1967, took an internship back in his hometown, but found himself faced with another pseudarthrosis by the end of that year. This time they fitted him with a full-body brace, which permitted him to be up and about after surgery, but the fusion did not heal. A sixth operation was performed out of state at a prestigious medical center leaving him with another full-body brace, this time with a halo attachment to his head so that he could return home and participate in a physical medicine and rehabilitation residency. Luckily, he had no pain and good function for the next three years and was able to walk only with the assistance of a cane and complete the last stages of his medical training. By 1975, however, back pain began again, but this time it affected his lower extremity function. X-ray films revealed that his spine had tilted 30° with osteoarthritis and bony spurs below L3. Another fusion relieved the radiating pain but unfortunately it did not heal; thus, an eighth operation was performed, but this time the surgeons insisted on a full-body cast and immobilization in bed again for the usual six months. When finally he went back to work, he began to use a wheelchair because of increasing fatigue. However, even with this assistance, it was becoming increasingly difficult to put in a full day's work. When he got home in the evenings, he was exhausted.

Bill married Susan, a nurse with whom he worked, in the late 1970s. This extraordinarily happy event offset the frustration of repeated surgery and of his inability to practice medicine without the interruptions caused by an uncooperative spine. He had two more operations to insert electrical stimulators in his back, which successfully stimulated bone growth. However, by this time, the many operations, the scar tissue, and the wear and tear all took their toll. By midmorning he was overcome by a pervasive exhaustion and had to lie down. Thus, the issue of retirement had to be faced. Although his colleagues had been exceedingly undemanding of him, they needed someone on whom they could count. In reality, at this point, he just did not have the energy to work even a half day. Consequently, in 1983, Bill retired from the active practice of medicine after less than nine years of post-residency work. He protests that if it had only been the pain problem, he could have kept working, but the fatigue made it literally impossible to continue. In addition to the pain and fatigue, Bill has recently noticed increasing weakness in certain leg muscles, which he thought had recovered from the polio completely. Hypertension has been a major problem since 1974 and seems to be unresponsive to the normal dosages of medication. Pain continues to be a problem, and he needs maintenance doses of pain medication daily also. Now he is at home, pacing himself in order to conserve his energy. Even going out to dinner or to the symphony is a major event that usually requires 24 hours of rest afterwards in order to continue some semblance of a normal life.

Always a very frugal person, Bill has lived very modestly, but comfortably, and has channeled a fair portion of his income into disability income insurance, a tax-deferred annuity, and investments. It is interesting to note that Bill had no trouble acquiring disability income insurance, whereas Jack found this to be impossible. Bill was displaying minimal evidence of disability at the time that the policy went into effect, since he was using only a cane. Also, perhaps his status as physician added credibility to his application and deferred some questions about previous disability problems. Currently, he, his wife, and daughter live adequately on disability income from two insurance policies and SSDI. The former two will provide income until he is 65, at which time he hopes that his retirement pension from the hospital, his tax-deferred annuity, and Social Security will cover his expenses. His medical expenses are still covered by insurance from the hospital for which he had worked and he is also covered by Medicare.

Bill, who is 51 now, occasionally wonders how his life would have turned out if he had not gotten polio. Would he have become a physician? He does not know, but probably not. College was not something that he considered seriously before the disability prevented him from automatically falling into the family pattern of getting some physically oriented work after graduation from high school. Why did he do it? Why did he become a physician when DVR's lack of encouragement was echoed by his family's concern about where the money would come from? He does not know. However, once he got the idea, it never occurred to him not to "go for it." His first orthopedic surgeon encouraged these aspirations and served as a wonderful role model even though he was not disabled himself. Nevertheless, despite the tremendous effort invested in his medical training and short-lived practice, Bill has no regrets. It has been a good life and he is glad that he could work as long as he did. Unfortunately, being a physician has not prevented or altered the physical course of the post-polio syndrome; nor has he had special entrée to magical information or interventions to halt the process of aging with a disability.

Currently, Bill spends his days reading, playing the piano, and participating in family and church activities. Although frustrated at times by his circumstances, life is not so bad, he claims. Since getting polio, he has spent so many hours, days, months, and even years flat on his back in bed that he knows how much worse life could be for him. Just being able to be up is a luxury for Bill and he takes nothing for granted.

Bill represents our polio survivors who have been pioneers, just as have those with spinal injury. Many have endured the bittersweet status of variable physical function: one day you have it, the next day you don't. Many have recovered sufficiently to blend anonymously into daily life with levels of stress, energy expenditure, and discomfort unrecognized by neighbors and co-workers. The toll for these physical options and freedoms is now being extracted as many face the onset of a second disability—severely compromised function reminiscent of their earlier days with polio. Bill had few environmental resources, but his intelligence and drive (and minimal level of disability in the early years) helped him to obtain an education that led to a high-paying professional job. Governmental help was crucial during medical school and without it he would not be a physician. Although he worked only nine years, his frugality and his eligibility for generous private benefits have given him a level of freedom not available to Sally, Jack, or Dave.

LISA

The Young Adult with Polio of Childhood Onset

Lisa experienced her first symptoms of the post-polio syndrome after only 20 years with the disability when her right thumb ceased to function while taking notes in a graduate school class. She was 22 years old at the time. Now she is 37.

Both Lisa and her mother, who was eight months pregnant with another child, came down with poliomyelitis at the same time. Luckily, her mother's case was so mild that she was not even hospitalized. Unfortunately for two-year-old Lisa, all of her extremities became totally paralyzed, including her respiratory function, and consequently she was placed in an iron lung and hospitalized for 16 months. Thankfully, her breathing returned to normal after six weeks, but, when she returned home, it was with leg braces, total paralysis from the waist down, only moderate muscle function in her left arm, and fairly good function in her right. The family had changed, however, in her absence. Her brother and sister had grown considerably since she had seen them last, and there was a new little sister whom she had never met.

This was the 1950s and a family of four children, one of whom was disabled, was a big financial responsibility for her engineer father. Therefore, when the hospital suggested that he could save money by buying her an adult-sized wheelchair, one she could grow into rather than replacing child-sized ones every few years, her father agreed. Thus, Lisa came home in a wheelchair that was so big that it would hold her and two additional children, and, of course, her short little arms could not reach the wheel rims. Consequently, she could never propel it by herself; she always had to ask for someone to push her.

Apparently, Lisa'a mother had always been "emotional," but now Lisa became the focus of much of her mother's hostility, although the rest of the family got a good share also. For example, mother decided that toileting Lisa was an intolerable burden; therefore, a schedule was established. Lisa could use the bedpan at 8:30 a.m., 1:00 p.m., and at bedtime. No more! If Lisa had an accident in between those times, mother would go into a rage. Because she was such a burden, Lisa would be given a bath only once every four months; a sponge bath once a week. Thus, within this atmosphere of animosity, Lisa's world was limited to her bed and the living room couch, with only occasional trips to the grocery store with mother. For diversion, Lisa watched TV and the squirrels that romped in the trees beside the house.

When she was seven, the issue of her schooling was discussed. The elementary school was only one block away and accessible by wheelchair, but the family did not think that education for a disabled person was necessary. Nevertheless, father believed that everyone ought to be able to read and write, even though he had no expectation that Lisa would ever lead an independent life, and thus he supported the idea of education. The school board, however, did not believe that a disabled child would be a good influence on the other children and consequently denied her admission. Fortunately, they authorized a tutor to come to the home three times a week for one hour and that became a highlight of Lisa'a week. It was also fun when some of the neighborhood children came to play with her, but mother viewed these visits as further burdens in her life. Thus, with all of her fussing and irritability, she made life miserable for everyone and gradually the children stopped coming.

Schooling was short-lived, however, because Lisa's spine had curved so profoundly from lack of proper bracing that her left lung collapsed. At this point, Lisa could hear her parents' arguments about what they should do with her.

The possibility of sending her to a hospital in Warm Springs, Georgia, that specialized in polio was discussed, but Lisa was afraid that they only wanted to get rid of her. Finally it was decided; she would go. Father drove her the 700 miles to the hospital, took her to the admissions office, and told her to be a good little girl as he left for the return drive home. Because the pediatric ward was full, Lisa was admitted to the teenager's ward, a seven-year-old among the big kids. It was lonely, frightening, and painful.

In order to straighten her spine, she was placed in a succession of body casts and also in splints because her arms and legs had developed contractions at the joints. After several painful months, however, the decision was made to surgically repair certain orthopedic deformities in her legs, which meant more pain and more casts. Finally, after eight months, Lisa was discharged to home with a complex schedule of procedures and considerable apparatus that added to her mother's perception of the unfair burden it was to have a disabled child.

While Lisa had been hospitalized, however, the family had moved out into the country to a house with six steps at the entrance and windows so high that one could not see out unless standing up, something Lisa could not do. The hospital dictated that she was to remain in a lying position for a total of 21 hours a day; uptime was limited to a maximum of three hours, two of which were spent hanging from a sling-like contraption that attached under her jaws; this was supposed to keep her head in proper alignment with her spine. When lying down during the day, she was placed in skeletal traction to keep her spine straight, and at night she slept in a Milwaukee brace. This apparatus looked somewhat like a bird cage around the upper part of her body, with metal rods and leather straps to keep her spine in alignment at night. Mother's temper constantly flared at Lisa and the whole family, and she frequently screamed at friends or even strangers in the store while pointing to Lisa, "You think you have it bad! Look what I have to put up with!" To make her life worse, the hospital had advised that she allow Lisa to use the bedpan at least 4 times a day.

Lisa was literally entombed in that house from the time she was seven until she was 16. A tutor came three times a week. Children did not visit, and her own brother and sisters tried to stay away from home as much as they possibly could to avoid the constant tension around the house. Mother was so unpredictable in her outbursts. One never knew what would set her off, and thus Lisa was constantly terrified of triggering her mother's anger. But dinnertime became a ritual of sadism. Everyone was expected to be in their seats at the table by 5:30 sharp. Mother would dish out food onto everyone's plate and all of the food had to be consumed before anyone was allowed to leave the table. Dinnertime was also used by mother as an occasion to discuss any misbehavior that had occurred during the previous 24-hour period, and, of course, this was just another opportunity to vent her anger on the whole family. Lisa reports today that it was not until six or seven years ago that she has been able to overcome her fear of middle-aged women and eating at a table with other people.

Books and television were Lisa's only solace. To cope with mother's tirades, she withdrew into herself and fantasized what the world might be like else-where. Television was helpful in that the sitcoms of the 1950s and 1960s, such as "Ozzie and Harriet" and "Leave It to Beaver," presented a more positive view of family life. Thus, she knew that everyone's life was not as bad as hers. However, Lisa wondered what possible purpose her life was meant to serve. She had no religious training, but, philosophically, even as a little girl, she had to come to terms with her daily agony. Thus, she grew to believe that her life had some meaning; she would make sure that she would help others some day, but she could not imagine how this would happen. Nevertheless, it was some-thing to believe in.

Intermittently over the years, she was sent back to Warm Springs for refitting of equipment or for additional surgery to correct some orthopedic problem. Each time that she returned home to her tomb the isolation, solitude, and terror seemed worse. Her older brother and younger sister were nice to her, but they tried to stay away from home as much as possible. Her father was essentially passive with regard to protecting the children from their mother's temper, but he too had his own ways of making life difficult. Basically, he ridiculed any-thing the children said, constantly telling them that they were silly or stupid. Thus, from their mother, the children learned fear; from their father, they learned self-doubt. Nevertheless, he emphasized education as a top priority in a child's life and placed strict demands that everyone get good grades. Lisa's older sister seemed to feel nothing but hate for all of the trouble that Lisa's dis-ability caused the family and sometimes Lisa could feel that the others con-curred. This was especially apparent when Lisa was 12 and the family was discussing a three-week vacation in California. Lisa was excited and asked to go to Disneyland. But as they planned the trip, they realized that Lisa with all of her equipment would be a great deal of trouble. Thus, the decision was made to drop her off at Warm Springs Hospital for an equipment fitting so that the family could have a real vacation on the West Coast. If there ever was a time that Lisa felt all alone, that was it. They brought her gifts when they returned and showed her pictures of all that they had seen. But she refused to look at them. The hurt was just too great to hide. The anger at all of these injustices was building within her but she dared not show it. She was only a child and she was trapped by her disability. All that she could do was to bide her time and that, indeed, would require four more years.

Finally, when she was 16 years old, life changed dramatically as the result of a return visit to Warm Springs. A friendly occupational therapist decided that Lisa should learn to do her own self-care and to use a more appropriate wheel-chair. The lessons challenged Lisa in ways that she had never thought possible before. The climax came when Lisa accomplished the feat of getting on and off the toilet by herself! No one who has gotten a Nobel Prize or Academy Award was happier or prouder of their achievement than Lisa because this was the beginning of freedom and the beginning of the rest of her life. No more sche-dules dictated by mother. Now she could bathe, dress, and go to the toilet whenever she wanted. All of her suppressed feelings seemed to give her a powerful drive to succeed—to take on every challenge that she could find. Thus, the self-confidence that this engendered spilled over to her social life and for the first time she was able to relate comfortably to the other kids her age in the hospital. She had her first boyfriend and experienced the camaraderie of teenage girls giggling about all of the things that kids do. For the first time she was a normal little girl.

Previously, the hospital personnel had viewed Lisa as a meek and passive little girl. But with the drive and determination that Lisa was now displaying, the counselors at the hospital prevailed on the family to let Lisa leave the house to go to high school. Luckily, the school board agreed to accept her. Thus, in her junior year, Lisa got out of her tomb, had an opportunity to relate to people on a normal everyday basis, and was determined to make every day count. She joined many extracurricular activities and tried to be just "one of the kids." Her classmates were very nice to her, but by the end of her senior year, Lisa realized that she had never been fully accepted. Never was she invited to their social events or parties after school. Everyone went to the prom but her. Thus, she started to get angry again. Life was not like it had been presented on television. Apparently, that was an idealized world that did not exist.

After high school graduation, father agreed to let her go to college. This meant going away from home for the first time, and it was rough. She had had only two years of "normal" living and consequently was hardly prepared for the independence and pressures of college, in a dormitory, with vast distances to cover in her wheelchair. Her grades suffered, and father was furious. Furthermore, her social life was a continuous series of disappointments, since she did not discriminate carefully as to which people would be good friends and which not. Thus, she got involved with some unpleasant people who treated her pretty badly. To make matters worse, many times she often went out on a blind date only to have the fellow barely conceal his annoyance at having to be with a woman in a wheelchair.

One man did not react that way. They became very good friends and in fact he avowed that he loved her and wanted to marry her. Danny was in a wheelchair himself as the result of spinal injury and he understood her as no one ever had before. She did not love him, but she was so grateful that he could love her that she agreed to marry him. Thanksgiving of her sophomore year, Danny and Lisa went to his home for the holidays and his family was very unhappy about the engagement. Thus, the tension was terrible and, after Lisa's own family experiences, she was devastated by the rejection that she felt from his parents too. One night, she overheard Danny and his father arguing about the proposed marriage, Danny's father yelling, "A man in a wheelchair has no business getting married, much less to another cripple!" During December, Danny began to drink heavily and finally after Christmas he broke off the engagement. She was depressed and barely made passing grades. Danny continued to drink and finally was killed in an auto accident. When Lisa found out, she became obsessed with the idea of her own death. She very carefully obtained the means to commit suicide, but she was never capable of carrying it out. A three-month counseling experience helped, but when the counselor was reassigned and could not see her anymore, her anger erupted and her attitude became "screw the world." And that is what she proceeded to do for the next several months. She hated everyone: nondisabled people, disabled people, everybody. The injustices that she had had to endure throughout her entire life flooded her with rage, and it was difficult to remember that her life was supposed to have some special meaning. But after several months, she cooled off, but not before she had challenged publicly every stereotype of disabled people. Today she can laugh at this, but then it was no laughing matter.

Lisa finished college and proceeded to graduate school to get a master's degree in rehabilitation counseling. The DVR had helped finance her undergraduate degree and now a stipend from the university supported her during her graduate training. However, early in her program, one of her professors called her into his office and said, "Lisa, there is such a terrible look of pain in your eyes. Is there something that I can do to help you?" Lisa broke into tears and poured out her life story. Thus began a counseling relationship of two years' duration that helped her to gain some perspective on her life and to establish the basis for making it into something special. All of that suffering had to be viewed as preparation for something better in life, and he helped her to mobilize the strength to continue to live. Of particular importance was his help in the matter of interpersonal relationships so that her future contacts with people were not so stormy and disappointing.

After graduation, Lisa decided to move to California. It seemed like a place of glamour, and, besides, now she could go independently to the places that her family visited on their vacation when she was 12 and left at the hospital. Lisa got an apartment and a job as an alcohol and drug abuse counselor and enjoyed life immensely. Within a few months she met an army sergeant, named David, who promptly fell in love with her and proposed marriage. Lisa was just beginning to experience a true freedom and did not want to settle down at this point, so she said no. Unfortunately, the agency for which she worked closed, and she could not find another job that she liked; consequently, she moved to another town. Work was no easier to find there either and money was running out. However, the last thing that she wanted to do was to call her parents for help, and thus when David came to visit and again proposed marriage, she accepted, but with some misgivings.

Two months after the marriage, the army sent David to Germany. Housing for dependents was difficult to find so, when she joined him, she found herself in a fourth floor apartment with no elevator. Entombed again, she got out of that place only three times, David having to carry her up and down four flights of stairs. Finally, he found a first floor apartment, but the cold, damp northern European weather was aggravating her respiratory function and she was constantly sick with pulmonary infections. Lisa had functioned on only one lung since age seven and now the infections debilitated her. The army sent them back to the States and he was stationed in the South. Lisa got a job as an alcohol and drug abuse counselor for the military and the years passed quietly. David retired from the army after 20 years, and they both moved back to California. David works as a salesman, Lisa as a disability rights counselor, and their salaries just barely meet expenses. His military pension covers the mortgage on their small house.

Lisa has spent the last several years becoming very active in the disability rights movement, in the post-polio support group effort, and in the independent living movement. Recently she won the Miss Wheelchair West competition, a second Nobel Prize or Academy Award for her. That evening, all dressed up on the stage, with her crown on and photographers snapping her picture, she heard someone say, "Oh, isn't she beautiful." Lisa turned around to see who they were talking about but no one was there. Suddenly she realized that they were talking about her. David was at her side as he has been throughout their marriage and Lisa remembered her childhood determination to make sure that her life would have some meaning. Now, as she has for years, Lisa is taking on the world with a vengeance. She hopes to educate "nondisabled" people about the rights and needs of those with disabilities. Also she hopes to help disabled people feel good about themselves and to learn to be assertive in facing the world. Certainly Lisa has done a masterful job of that herself.

When one meets Lisa, one sees a vibrant, charming, assertive, and intelligent woman. Never would one expect such a traumatic personal life history as the one just described. Surely she still has deep feelings about how she was treated in her earlier years, but she has gone beyond that and not allowed it to drag her down. Not surprisingly she has little to no contact with her family, but David has become her family now. Unfortunately, at age 37, Lisa is greatly worried about the progress of her post-polio symptoms. The first symptom occurred when she was 22 in college taking notes in class when her right thumb gave out. She has had to learn a new finger position for holding a pencil or pen. Her right arm, her good one, is getting weaker each year, and her scoliosis has become a problem again. In 1979, a spinal fusion was performed that has successfully reduced her spinal curvature, but her respiratory function is deteriorating yearly. Apparently, her thoracic muscles are becoming weaker, and, because of lack of proper oxygenation at night during sleep, her physician wants to do a permanent tracheostomy so that she can use a respirator at night. She refuses and has finally found a pulmonary specialist who agrees that there are many other avenues to try before such a drastic step is necessary. With an ironic laugh, Lisa told me the good news of finding such an understanding and knowledgable physician. The bad news is that this physician is not covered by her Blue Cross Preferred Provider Plan, and, thus, she will have to pay a large share of the costs out of her own pocket.

Over the years, Lisa has had surgery for bilateral carpal tunnel syndrome (pinched nerve in the wrist from years of transferring and wheelchair propulsion) and tennis elbow. Switching to an ultralight wheelchair has helped as has an electrically powered cartop wheelchair carrier. Now she is contemplating an electric wheelchair because of reduced function in her right arm and because of declining respiratory reserves.

Despite all of this, Lisa continues to be the dynamic and determined disability rights advocate who is working desperately to educate the public about the needs of people with disabilities and the experiences of a generation of people with polio residuals who are now experiencing problems that few professionals are prepared to handle. Thus, without a doubt, Lisa's life has had special meaning because she continues to be a major source of support to a large number of people who are feeling all alone with their post-polio symptoms.

Lisa's life as a child is hopefully not typical of how most children with disabilities are treated by their families, but, unfortunately, it happens more often than we realize. While there was no excuse for her mother's behavior, the onset of a disability is a major stress event for the entire family, and this must become a focus for rehabilitation interventions by the entire team. The siblings and parents experience problems with the disability as does the disabled child, and, thus, family relationships need to be a constant consideration throughout the childhood period.

Even though Lisa is only 37 years old, she is experiencing the problems of aging with a disability. It seems that this aging problem is not so much an issue of chronological age but one of length of time with the disability. In Lisa's case, the initial polio episode was very severe; she has been left with significant physical impairment; and she has lived a very active life since she was able to get out of her home. Most of the persons with major physical disabilities who are experiencing aging problems are in the older age groups, but as we explore this issue in the remainder of the book, we must not forget that those who acquired polio as children may be vulnerable to these symptoms even after 20 years with the disability.

THE PENALTY OF DISABILITY

These biographies represent a diversity of lifestyles, backgrounds, personalities, and environmental resources, but they have one thing in common: the disability imposed a penalty that reduced their freedoms. Throughout their lives, they have been penalized emotionally, physically, and financially, yet they have survived because of an indomitable human spirit. They have the will to live and the determination to accept responsibility for their own lives. Living with a disability is physically demanding, emotionally frustrating, and financially depleting, but each of these people has lived a useful life and has had accomplishments and failures, happiness and unhappiness. Consequently, by all standards, these are "normal" people who just happen to have a physical impairment that requires a greater energy expenditure to accomplish most daily activities and greater monthly expense just to survive.

In each case, the presence of the physical disability has deprived the person of options—of certain freedoms regarding how one will live one's life. Two of our biographees have been "compensated" for their loss of freedoms, one through the federal government and one through an insurance program mandated by the government. Let us note, as Frank has said, that there is no amount of money that makes living with a disability something that one would elect to do if there was a choice. The other six have been penalized with no compensation. Two, Clifford and Bill, were able to achieve high incomes through advanced education, which has helped them to overcome the financial penalty of disability, at least up to the present. But Sally, Jack, and Dave have been further penalized by our fragmented social legislation, which was not intended to keep people poor but which requires that they remain so if they expect any assistance. These three have not been able to overcome the lack of environmental support despite deep personal commitments on their parts to self-reliance and financial independence. Thus, there are inequities in how we treat people with disabilities that are difficult to justify in a democratic society supposedly based on the principles of freedom and equality of opportunity.

Now after a lifetime of struggle, these people are aging and the physical penalty is increasing. Unfortunately, this increases the personal and financial penalty (costs) exponentially so that each of our resourceful individuals is deeply worried about the future. *Let there be no doubt that as these individuals age, each of them emphasizes one thing: as their function declines, they want to remain free— free to manage their own lives in their own homes. No one mentioned the need to build more nursing homes as a solution to the issue of aging with a physical disability.*

Death is a part of life, aging is a form of growth, and these processes should be viewed within the context of health. All of our biographees are healthy. They may have physical limitations and declining function, but these are normal features of everyone's life across the decades and thus should not be considered to be sicknesses. Consequently, it is necessary to establish a conceptual framework for our study of aging and disability—a framework that views life to be the process of achieving a harmony among psychosocial (P), biological–organic (O), and environmental (E) influences and health to be the optimum balance among these three variables.

3

Health and Physical Disability

HEALTH AS A BALANCING ACT

Each of us "knows" what health is; we "know" that it is more than the absence of disease; we "know" that many inner and outer events (stresses) influence our well-being and health. This "knowing" consists of a deep intuitive sense and understanding, the kind of understanding that unfortunately is often suspect in our technologically oriented society. Thus, we sometimes distrust this knowledge and look outside of ourselves for answers, answers that we mistakenly assume are synonymous with the accumulation of facts. Unfortunately, the history of science demonstrates repeatedly that the facts of today are often discredited tomorrow. Therefore, in what can we believe? Where can we find consistency in a rapidly changing world? It seems to me that what we really need is a philosophy, or a conceptual framework if you prefer, which presents a coherent set of beliefs or ideas that forms the basis for a course of action, even though we recognize that the facts do change and will change. It is interesting to note that, although we know what health is, we rarely stop to examine this concept and, as a result, ignore the absence of an explicit philosophy of health care in our western society. Therefore, this chapter explores the concept of health and attempts to outline a philosophy that applies to all health care, and particularly to health care of an aging and disabled population.

Health is based on a balance of biological, psychological, and environmental forces that allows an equilibrium, i.e., homeostasis, to exist. Although equilibrium may give the appearance of rest, it is, rather, a dynamic process based on adaptation to constant change. There are many elements and forces within the human being and environment that, in essence, form an elaborate system of interchange and flux. The human body itself is constantly evolving, generating new cells, and discarding old ones, and the environment is repeatedly presenting us with challenge and stress. Thus, despite this fluctuating human-environment system, equilibrium is achieved most of the time, and most of us mind-bodies are healthy most of the time.

44

Some definitions of health imply wholeness and perfection, but how many of us are truly whole and which of us are perfect? Such concepts of wholeness and perfection seem static and arbitrary and imply an all or nothing phenomenon that would exclude practically everyone. If you lose a finger, are you no longer whole and therefore unhealthy? If you have a scar on your face, are you imperfect and therefore unhealthy? If you have a spinal injury or the residuals of polio, are you by definition unhealthy? Individuals with physical disabilities are subject to the same counterbalancing forces and stresses as everyone else and, therefore, are as able to be healthy or unhealthy as "nondisabled" people. The point to emphasize is that biological or organic influences are only one factor in the equation, in the balancing act leading to health. The personal, spiritual, and environmental influences in one's life have a similar influence on health and are part of the balancing act that we all perform every day.

Weil (1983), a physician, believes that there are a variety of treatment approaches that have been established to treat sickness and promote health, and he offers the following principles of health and illness relevant to the topic of living and aging with a physical disability.

Perfect health is not attainable. The balancing act of health implies change, subtle and gross, hourly and yearly. Change is the essence of life and our bodies are constantly changing within the context of our fluctuating psychological state and environmental pressures. Thus, we cannot expect to attain some absolute level of perfect health that is static and never-changing.

It is all right to be sick. Viewing sickness as a calamity and misfortune, rather than as one cycle in the process of achieving equilibrium, arouses negative emotions that hinder healing and adaptation rather than promote them. Anger, guilt, and anxiety about being sick create a psychological climate that impedes the body's natural ability to heal.

The body has innate healing abilities. Healing comes from the inside, not outside, as the eight biographies in Chapter 2 aptly demonstrate. It is the human spirit that restores equilibrium, and this equilibrium does not derive from external agents. As any perceptive physician knows or learns, the art of healing involves the arousal of the person's will to live and his or her active participation in the treatment process.

Agents of disease are not causes of disease. Agents of disease (viruses, bacteria, noxious pollutants, potential sources of trauma, etc.) are all around us, but most of us do not develop symptoms until our internal state becomes unbalanced and we become susceptible to these agents. "A person solidly equilibrated in a phase of relative health can often interact with these agents and not get sick. Since internal factors determine the nature of our relationships with them, the true causes of disease are internal" (Weil, 1983, p. 56). Cousins' (1979) description of the circumstances leading up to his life-threatening illness beautifully illustrates this point.

All illness has a psychological component. All of us are mind-bodies, each totally interpenetrates the other, and there is absolutely no way that you can separate the two. To treat bodies without regard for the mind is the height of arrogance and the depth of ignorance. To say that an illness has a psychological component has been used by some professionals in a derogatory sense and with the implication that the illness is not real, is less important, and, therefore, is not to be considered seriously. We, unfortunately, have all too readily bought into this belief in an attempt to protest, "But it is real; it is important; it should be taken seriously; and of course it is physical." Thus, a mechanical approach to diagnosis and treatment has dehumanized illness so that physician and patient participate in this "folie a deux" (mutually reinforcing craziness) that organic-bodily variables can be treated without regard for the person experiencing the problem or the environmental factors contributing to it.

Subtle manifestations of illness precede gross ones. It is easier to treat problems before they become major and, thus, each person needs to learn to listen to the internal rhythm and signals of the body and to notice subtle changes. People with long-term physical disability learn this technique exquisitely well and it accounts for their longevity. This entails accepting responsibility for their own lives and participating in the decision-making regarding the timing and nature of intervention strategies. Unfortunately, our current practices and procedures do not encourage this approach, since reimbursement for care is often tied to "legitimate diagnoses" (major problems) and many professionals do not trust reports of subjective findings in the absence of quantifiable problems.

Every body is different. Every person is unique; we all vary tremendously even though superficially we are the same. Thus, it is impossible to plan a life-style, a treatment strategy, or a program that is suitable for all. Patterns of growth, function, and aging will vary depending on the inherent differences in bodies and in mind-bodies. As a result, a highly individualized approach to assessment and treatment is mandatory.

Every body has a weak point. To identify one's weak points may allow a person to detect early signs of imbalance in health in order to institute remedial or preventive measures immediately. In addition, over the years we may find that there is one body system that is the focus of intermittent problems or dysfunction with age. Thus, diversity and heterogeneity will be obvious across the life span and across people, even among those united under one label, such as spinal cord injury, post-polio, etc.

Consequently, aging is a part of living and it need not imply bad health, sickness, or disability. Rather, it is part of the balancing act in which we have all participated since birth. In fact, literally, aging starts at birth and occurs throughout the life span; thus, there is no definable starting point for aging, nor is there a definable date on which one becomes aged. It is interesting to note that even within the field of gerontology, there is not unanimity of opinion as to what constitutes the process of aging (Blumenthal, 1983). However, a recent conference entitled "Modern Biological Theories of Aging" revealed that, although there are a variety of theories on the causes of aging, these theories agree that aging results from the cumulative damages to organs, cells, or molecules over the course of life. But whether future research will be able to alter the progress of aging or only treat some of the diseases associated with the later years remains to be seen (*New York Times*, June 10, 1986). Therefore, let us focus on health and the variety of influences that must be kept in equilibrium in order to be healthy.

THE PARTICIPANTS IN THE BALANCING ACT

Behavior (B) or health is a function of the interaction of psychosocial (P), biological–organic (O), and environmental (E) influences:

$$B = f(P,O,E)$$

Table 3-1 presents a catalogue of variables that interact and influence all of our lives (disabled and "nondisabled"), and the dynamic balance among these variables is a major factor in determining health status at any one moment. When thinking about health, there is a tendency to review the list of organic (O) factors first (but this is thinking about sickness, not health) and then to become overwhelmed by the sheer number of psychosocial (P) and environmental (E) variables listed, decide it is impractical to deal with such complexity, and proceed to focus exclusively on the biological–organic factors. It is important to realize that this approach, used for the last 100 years in western medicine, has resulted in what is essentially a sickness treatment system rather than a health care system. This approach has led to the body being considered as

Table 3-1. *Behavior (B) as a Function of the Interaction of Psychosocial (P), Organic (O), and Environmental (E) Variables*

Psychosocial variables (P)	Organic variables (O)	Environmental variables (E)
Take responsibility for self	Intelligence and cognitive	Income
Will to live	ability	Transportation
Social skills	Endurance	Architectural and geo-
Style of coping with stress	Strength	graphic barriers
Locus of control (I-E)	Perceptual motor coordi-	Access to knowledgable
Self-confidence	nation	health professionals
Judgment	Aptitudes	Educational and vocational
Problem-solving ability	Amount of physical im-	resources
Education	pairment	Financial disincentives
Work history	Sensory abilities	Family and interpersonal
Job skills	Bladder and bowel control	support
Cultural and ethnic group	Respiratory function	Socioeconomic status
Gender	Pain	Availability of physical
Creativity	General health status	assistance (if needed)
		Behavioral supervision (if needed)
		Payment for medical care
		Role models

separate from the mind, to be treated as if it were a machine to be "fixed." It has also led to an overemphasis on objective data and the devaluation of subjective data, and to an over-reliance on technology and a decline in emphasis on the art of healing.

The psychosocial variables (P) include all of the intrinsic characteristics that might be subsumed under the construct of personality. Yet, it is more than the intrapsychic features that are important here. The person's work history, education, and cultural-ethnic experiences are integral elements of the person but also are aspects of the environment as well. The organic (O) or biological variables include those body and mental functions that derive from genetic, environmental, and behavioral lifestyle influences. Rather than being static, these organic variables will vary according to our age, health, and general well-being. The environmental (E) variables are those factors distal to the person that determine whether or not a physical impairment will become a handicap in achieving health, well-being, and productivity. These variables will be assets or liabilities to function and, thus, are critical parameters in the feedback loop among P, O, and E variables. Because the human being is a complex whole, a system, none of the above variables can truly be considered to be separate and uninfluenced by the entire equation.

No matter whether one is disabled or "nondisabled," successful and healthy living in our society entails at least three major categories of activities or behavior (B) (Table 3-2). The first category includes survival activities: the promotion of wellness, avoidance of medical complications, and performance of the usual activities of daily living. If the person is not capable of physical independence, the person can and must accept responsibility for ensuring that these matters are taken care of properly by someone else. Our biographies demonstrate how critical this is to successful adjustment to a physical disability. The second category, harmonious living, includes all of the social skills that promote a stable environment for living, working, and socializing. This category of function is critical to successful living with a disability because one so often needs to rely on the goodwill of "nondisabled" persons. Therefore, the ability to generate this goodwill can powerfully influence the harmony and equilibrium of one's life, especially for those with quadriplegia. Productivity, the third category, entails more than employment but includes all of those activities that contribute to a sense of usefulness and satisfaction with life. Essentially, these are the reasons for living, the reasons for getting out of bed each morning. When these decline in number, the human system will go out of balance very quickly. Consequently, among these three categories there is an interaction. Severely curtailed survival activities will have an unsettling effect on one's satisfaction with life and productivity. Equally obvious, if one feels unproductive, unneeded, and useless, if one has no real reason for getting out of bed each morning, there is less reason to take care of one's body. Thus, how one performs these activities (B) is influenced by the P,O,E interaction, which in turn influences the P, O, and E variables. *As a result, our behavior is a part of our*

Table 3-2. *Behavioral Components of Health (B)*

Survival activities
   Promotion of wellness
   Prevention of medical problems
   Activities of daily living (bathing, grooming, dressing, eating)
   Housekeeping
   Mobility

Harmonious living and working environment
   Family relationships
   Friendships
   Relations with service personnel and co-workers
   Relations to authority figures
   Financial management
   Management of personal affairs

Productivity
   Employment in or out of the home
   Educational activities
   Family and social roles
   Community service
   Avocations
   Scholarly pursuits
   Artistic endeavors
   Athletic endeavors

system and not only reflects our health status but determines significant aspects of our health status.

This is the meaning of a system, a mind-body system. You can fractionate and analyze it only for discussion purposes, but in actuality the whole is more than the sum of its parts. *We have ignored the concepts of wholeness and system in our western medical treatment and deceive ourselves that true understanding comes from analyzing the body into its component parts in order to understand how it works.* On the contrary, you can never understand a system by fragmentation and analysis alone. Unless you put the parts back into the context of the system, there is no understanding, no true knowledge, only a collection of facts without coherence or unity.

SICKNESS TREATMENT VERSUS HEALTH CARE

Western science has made tremendous advances in the last 200 years in examining the physical world and the more mechanical operations of the human body. At the same time, however, we have failed to develop a coherent philosophy that unites our information into a framework that serves as a guide for its use. The scientific method emphasizes analytical thinking, quantitative measurements, and objective data in order to explore *how* things work, not *why* things work as they do. So much information has been amassed regarding human biology that the body has been fragmented into organ systems, and medical specialties have been created in order to focus on one segment of human function, unfortunately in isolation from the rest of the body. While the scientific method has been responsible for great advances that have saved the lives of many people, it has subtly been used to define the nature of reality. This mistake has unintentionally brought suffering to many people as a result of a mechanical, impersonal approach to treatment (Cassell, 1976). We have all too frequently lost sight of the human as a dynamic, spiritual entity that cannot be fragmented for quantification, analysis, and transformation into strictly objective data.

In the last 50 years, there has been a transformation in the field of medicine that has extended the lives of many people, disabled and "nondisabled." None of these advances is intrinsically bad, wrong, or intentionally harmful, but *the problem lies in the imbalance in approach* based on the lack of a coherent philosophy of human life as an integral part of the natural environment. Rene Descartes, Francis Bacon, and Isaac Newton not only established the conceptual framework for the scientific revolution but divorced science from philosophy and religion, which, with the aid of the industrial revolution, has established our current set of assumptions about the study of man, nature, and man's relationship to nature. This is essentially a mechanistic approach to science, to medicine, and to our relationship with the environment. However, the most prestigious of all sciences, physics, has come to realize that the world and its components cannot be viewed only mechanistically and be analyzed in isolation from the context in which it occurs or is being studied (Zukav, 1979). Rather, our universe must be viewed as a dance of energy components, mutually interacting, and the observer and the observed are part of the same interactive system. Quantum physics has made discoveries that the other branches of science have chosen to ignore because these discoveries challenge the very premises on which the other branches of science operate: analysis, reductionism, and quantification are the only legitimate approaches to reality that traditional science recognizes (Capra, 1982).

Unfortunately, this attitude is apparent in many of our approaches to medicine. For example, many professionals believe that, if it cannot be measured, it is not important, and if it cannot be proven by the scientific method, it does not exist. Consequently, we have a sickness treatment system, a system that focuses on demonstrable biological–organic (O) dysfunction (pathology) in isolation from the human being (P,O,E) participating in that function, a system that lacks any coherent philosophy of health, a system with no true respect for, nor understanding of, the wholeness and balance that is entailed in life. In actuality, sickness is only a symptom of lack of health, a symptom of an imbalance somewhere in our elaborate feedback loop, but we delude ourselves that medication, surgery, or some technological intervention directed at only a biological–organic (O) dysfunction will completely solve the problem. Rather, health and cure of sickness derive from a restoration of the balance of mind-body-environment (P,O,E).

Table 3-3 describes some features of a sickness treatment versus health care

Table 3-3. *Comparison of Two Models of Treatment*

Sickness treatment system	Health care system
Acute orientation	Acute and chronic orientation
Analysis into parts	Synthesis of parts into whole
Fragmented approach	Systems approach
Objective data only	Objective and subjective data
Crisis intervention	Problem prevention
Professional is source of knowledge	Professional and patient are both sources of knowledge
Psychological component considered abnormal	Psychological component considered to be normal
Little coordination of services	Services coordinated by a "case manager"
Physician is gatekeeper to all services	Equal access to a variety of services
Hospital and clinic focus	Community focus
Person is passive recipient of services	Person is active participant in health process
Focus on organic variables almost exclusively	Focus on psychological, organic, environment interaction

system that help to elucidate this very complex topic. In a system oriented to treating sickness, there is a tendency to focus on treating acute episodes of an illness and to devote few resources to preventing complications and the comprehensive management of chronic illness or disability. However, both acute and chronic care are emphasized in a health-oriented system. With the sickness approach, the operational premise is that the body (O) is best managed by analyzing its component parts, and diagnostic efforts are directed toward determining which part needs treatment; it basically is a fragmented approach to health care. A health care system emphasizes the inherent unity of all body parts, and special steps are taken to integrate all diagnostic data into an "environmental impact report," so to speak, in order to assess the implications of treatment on the whole body system (P,O,E). Furthermore, the health care approach is based on the premise that people do have some intuitive, subjective knowledge about their own bodies, which is valuable information, essential to the evaluation and treatment process, whereas, in the sickness treatment approach, objective, quantifiable information is preferred and trusted implicitly. As a result, the sickness treatment system operates in a crisis intervention mode, not the problem prevention mode of a true health care system.

In the sickness treatment approach, professionals (physicians, psychologists, therapists) are frequently considered to be the repository of all knowledge about health and sickness. With this role has come an allied one of protecting the public from misinformation and ministrations not approved by or supervised by these professionals. (However, all professional licensing is aimed at guarding a field of practice, partly to protect the public and partly to protect the incomes of the professionals involved.)

In the sickness treatment system, any hint of a psychological component to an illness leads to the question of the "reality" of the illness. Yet, in a health care system, all illness is believed to be real, and all illness is expected to have a psychological component, unless the person is dead. Stress is a part of life; stress influences health and sickness; stress is present whenever one does not feel well. Another key feature of a sickness treatment system is the focus on hospital or clinic for the delivery of all services, whereas sickness and health must also be treated in the environment in which a person lives. Thus, home health care and independent living programs are a wonderful step in bridging the gap between sickness treatment and health care.

As an example of how these two systems might approach the same problem, let us consider a pressure sore problem. If a quadriplegic's car is stolen and there is no insurance to replace it, the lack of transportation leads to the loss of the job and income. The person feels useless and unproductive at home, becomes depressed, develops disturbances of sleep and appetite, which lead to lowered energy and endurance. Under these circumstances, he is less likely to seek alternative avenues of productivity, which guarantees a continued loss of income, increased family stress, and the wife deciding to seek employment. This reduces her availability to serve as a personal care attendant, which, in addition to all of the above, results in a pressure sore on his buttocks. The typical intervention strategy in the sickness treatment system consists of lectures on the importance of relieving skin pressure along with surgery and/or immobilization to heal the pressure sore. In a health care system, however, the intervention strategy would consist of assisting with new transportation arrangements, assisting him with job hunting, surgery and/or immobilization to heal the pressure sore, monitoring the depression, encouraging him to become fully productive again, and perhaps counseling for the family.

Thus, our three categories of activities (survival, harmonious living, and productivity) are behavioral manifestations of a healthy state. An imbalance, i.e., problems in one or more of the psychosocial (P), biological–organic (O), and environmental (E) areas, will alter our performance of these activities in subtle and not so subtle ways. Change may occur immediately and dramatically or slowly and subtly. The development of a pressure sore in the example used above is the end result of a gradually growing imbalance that began with the loss of vital transportation. More dramatic events, such as autonomic dysreflexia, a kidney infection, or the death of a spouse, have a more immediate impact on function and behavior. Because a large proportion of the dramatic issues derive from a sudden imbalance in a biological–organic (O) variable, there is a tendency to believe that these are the only important variables that need to be considered.

IMPLICATIONS FOR REHABILITATION

In the 1940s and 1950s, there was a new population of persons in the western world: those who had not died of major illness or injury and would live as disabled people. Thus, the opportunity to implement a true health care model arose. It was believed that, although these people could not be cured, they need not and should not be allowed to die or just be warehoused in custodial facilities. Consequently, Donald Munro, Howard Rusk, Ernest Bors, Ludwig Guttmann, William Spencer, Justus Lehmann, Frederick Kottke, and many others pioneered the field of rehabilitation medicine to help disabled people live functional and satisfying lives outside of hospitals, in their own homes with their families. At the same time, the medical sciences were making rapid advances based on research into organic factors and the development of new diagnostic technology. Research in these areas was federally financed and largely based in university medical schools.

With such an emphasis on the pursuit of control over organic variables in order to cure disease or to prevent it, rehabilitation was frequently viewed as a low-prestige specialty. It did not focus on new discoveries leading to cures or on the development of new procedures that "solved" problems, as did specialties such as surgery, cardiology, radiology, and oncology. Departments with a heavy biological research focus became exceedingly powerful in medical schools and hospitals. Large amounts of federal money were available, but to obtain it generally meant emphasizing basic science research that fractionated the body into smaller and smaller units. Naturally, there was pressure within the field of medical rehabilitation to compete. Unfortunately, within many medical schools today, research that focuses on practical issues such as helping disabled people lead more satisfactory lives may be considered "weak science," with more prestige attached to cellular, molecular, and biological research, i.e., "hard science." As a result, since the late 1940s there has been increasing pressure to adopt the operational policies and orientation of the sickness treatment system despite the original ideals for the field. While there are notable exceptions, both in program leaders and programs, the overall trend has been toward acute disability management and biologically oriented research in order to survive as a field. There are many caring physicians in rehabilitation who feel this schizophrenia on a daily basis but have felt forced to play the game in order to demonstrate the concepts of rehabilitation. This approach has been encouraged by federal programs that set guidelines for research and demonstration grants that emphasize accountability, measurability, and objectivity in data collection. These are all worthy goals but more easily applied to organic variables. Consequently, reality is defined only in terms of what can be measured, and organic factors have become the predominant reality in our medical system.

Yet, key physicians and other rehabilitation professionals have participated with federal program officers in defining the content of research programs and the guidelines for evaluation. Thus, we have a mutually reinforcing system of well-intentioned specialists and well-intentioned federal officials whose design of the field of rehabilitation reflected what they sincerely believed to be best. So rehabilitation medicine continues to focus on acute management of the new disability while becoming increasingly estranged from the long-term and broader health needs of disabled people. While there was a practical and political necessity to shape the programs in this manner to justify funding, rehabilitation has not been able to demonstrate its strengths but rather has had to emulate the weaknesses of an imbalanced approach to people's lives. Some professionals will feel unjustifiably attacked by this analysis, and others will admit that they feel the schizophrenia but have perceived no way out. One physician friend, chairman of a university department of rehabilitation medicine, has admitted to me privately that he could never reveal the depth of his interest in broader health issues without a loss of prestige with his colleagues. Because of his position, he must play the game of basic science research, acute medical management, grantsmanship, and power politics of the federal-state rehabilitation system in order to survive. He is an honest man, a caring physician, and his program is an outstanding one, albeit within the traditional system.

As a result, we have a system in which the programs are designed by the very people who will benefit from them in terms of professional power, prestige, and income. *Unfortunately, the input of people with disabilities is solicited only occasionally, and even though many centers have consumer advisory panels, these groups have no authority to shape programs or allocate resources.* Disabled people have little say in what services will be offered by a rehabilitation center, since very few centers have even asked clients what they need and want. We professionals determine what disabled people need. Consumers have little say as to what will be the content of research into the nature or course of their disabilities. We professionals who are not experiencing those disabilities determine what needs to be studied. Now, no one would propose that disabled people without professional and scientific training are fully qualified to define the total program of research nationally. Yet, we professionals with scientific training but without the experience of living with the disability feel fully qualified to plan such programs. Isn't this a double standard? Thus, the gap between the needs of the population of persons with disability who are aging and the programs in existence nationally is widening and many rehabilitation professionals are unaware of this. We all go to professional conferences and participate in our annual self-congratulation sessions in which we reassure ourselves that we are advancing the state of the art. But who defines the state of the art? Thus, we professionals often operate within a realm that greatly differs from the reality that is lived by person with disabilities, and because of our *social* isolation from people with disabilities, we seldom realize how wide the schism is.

The field of psychology, too, has been seduced by the sickness treatment model. Despite our supposed concern for the whole person, concepts of mental "illness" dominate the field and many in the new specialty of health psychology, for example, are carving up the person into component parts for analysis and research with the same finesse many physicians do. History repeats itself as health psychology becomes the favored child, while rehabilitation psychology is viewed as an ugly stepchild. In order to be considered scientific, much research in the behavioral sciences has been located in laboratory settings and has focused on quantifiable data that can be replicated; unfortunately, this has occurred at the expense of research into the broader issues of people functioning in complex natural environments. Consequently, psychologists have concentrated almost exclusively on the psychosocial (P) variables, physicians and others have focused on the biological (O) variables, and only a small percentage of professionals of any specialty have focused on the human as a P,O,E system.

Now for the other side of the picture. The evolution of our sickness treatment medical establishment has placed many physicians, federal program officers, and other professionals under tremendous pressure to conform to the system while attempting to implement a systems model of rehabilitation. With all of the glamour attached to the saving of lives, many dedicated professionals have persisted in fighting for services to those whose lives have been saved. Consequently, the medical management of disability today is spectacularly different from what it was in the 1940s and 1950s, and therefore, it is truly amazing how far rehabilitation has come since that time. Furthermore, rehabilitation has pioneered the multidisciplinary approach to treatment even though true interdisciplinary working relationships have not been fully realized in some settings. Currently, many rehabilitation centers have developed a wide array of services to help the newly disabled person integrate into the community, although these services do not seem to be widely available to those with long-term disability. Recently, the National Council on the Handicapped has been initiated to provide input to federal programs regarding the needs of those with disabilities. Unfortunately, the council has no authority to shape programs or to allocate funds, and consequently, its role is advisory. Now with the concern about costs of health care, rehabilitation as a multidisciplinary, P,O,E systems approach to disability is even more vulnerable to the pervasiveness of the sickness treatment model. While the field of rehabilitation may not have fully realized as true a health care and systems model as it could, those advances it has made are now threatened with elimination.

This pattern of professionals determining what services will be given, what research will be conducted, what type of training will be given is not unique to the rehabilitation field but is characteristic of how the American medical establishment, encouraged by the federal government, has evolved since World War II (Lewis and Sheps, 1983; Starr, 1982). Furthermore, in today's business climate in which medicine is practiced and sickness treated, many professionals or hospitals have not truly asked what patients and families want, what services they need, how they would like these services "delivered." Rather, it is increasingly the issue of costs and profits that determines the range, depth, and quality of sickness treatment given.

IS PROFIT COMPATIBLE WITH GOOD HEALTH CARE?

In any discussion of a sickness treatment approach versus a health care approach, the issue of profit needs to be addressed. *Is it morally right to profit from someone's sickness?* It is striking that this question is not asked very frequently. In fact, it is interesting how infrequently the terms "right" and "wrong" are used today. Pragmatism reigns supreme, and the resulting questions become, "Does it work?" "Does it make money?" Furthermore, these questions lead to an emphasis on the short term, since long-term planning often involves the reduction of immediate profits.

We all deserve to make a reasonable income based on an exchange of services for dollars, or services for goods, or services for services. But profit is that amount that can be garnered beyond the costs of giving the service and achieving a reasonable income. (Please, let us not quibble as to the definition of reasonable.) Making money and amassing profit have become so much a part of the American way of life it seems almost unpatriotic to raise *questions about the total applicability of this concept to all areas of human existence.* Certainly, the success and advances of the western countries, America in particular, in the last 200 years have been based on the principles of freedom, individualism, and free enterprise. However, with every right goes a responsibility; with the right to make a profit goes the responsibility to give maximum quality or full and satisfactory service. People are very concerned about protecting their rights. Perhaps they should give equal attention to carrying out their responsibilities. Consequently, it is important to emphasize that I do not intend to endorse the concept of socialism nor socialized medicine, but I do intend to raise the question as to whether the motivation to make a profit is compatible with the motivation to give good care to sick, old, or disabled people.

The American medical establishment has fought consistently to maintain a free enterprise system for their services (Starr, 1982), and now hospitals and corporations have decided to cash in on this "business" (Wohl, 1984; Califano, 1986). Unfortunately, the whole concept of a sickness treatment system feeds naturally into the format of a business venture in which units of treatment can be given to parts of the body. The body is a machine; the hospital is a repair facility; and we have a variety of technically oriented personnel that are trained to examine, service, and repair various parts. As with an airplane, we have our engine specialists, our fuselage specialists, our hydraulic specialists, and our electronic specialists. If something cannot be fixed, we even have repair by replacement using organic or mechanical parts.

Prior to 1983, third-party payers (insurance companies or the government) would be billed for any services or repairs deemed appropriate by the physician and costs shot up to 11% of the gross national product. When you take a human system and give services and repairs primarily to the biological–organic (O) variables and ignore the P,O,E interaction, costs go up because you may not be treating the major systems problems or you may be treating only fragments of the body and inadvertently producing side-effects in other parts of the system. It is not unusual to have as many as 11 different medical specialists involved with a seriously ill person in an intensive care unit. Each physician treats his or her assigned part of the body and often no *one* physician truly functions as a *program manager*, although there will be one primary physician for the medical record. Unfortunately, complications may multiply as each specialist treats one body part and these interventions impinge on the rest of the body. Furthermore, the patient's family is on an emotional roller coaster depending on which medical specialist they talked to most recently.

Since 1983, the DRG (diagnostic related groups) concept has been applied to Medicare and has been adopted by many other third-party payers, so that a predetermined fee for fixing any one of 468 different physical repair problems (diagnoses) is given to the hospital. Now there is concern that people are not getting all of the services that they need because the hospital needs to discharge them *before* their DRG fee is reached *in order to* make a profit. Consequently, the DRG concept is a natural byproduct of a sickness treatment system that has been more and more obviously fueled by a desire for profit.

Hilfiker (1986), a physician, states:

> Private medicine is abandoning the poor. As a family doctor practicing in the inner city of Washington, I am embarrassed by my profession's increasing refusal to care for the indigent; I am angry that the poor are being shuttled to inferior public clinics and hospitals for their medical care (p. 44).

He goes on to discuss the complex nature of the practice of medicine today that has led to this situation.

> But the cause that is probably most obvious to the lay public but singularly invisible to the medical community: medicine is less and less rooted in service and more and more based in money. Physicians are too seldom servants and too often entrepreneurs. A profitable practice has become primary. The change has been so dramatic and so far reaching that most of us do not even recognize that a transformation has taken place, that there might be an alternative. We simply take it for granted that economic factors will be primary even for the physician. While we physicians have been unable or unwilling to recognize this increasing monetarization of our work, society seems to have perceived it clearly and reacted in kind (pp. 45–46).

Not all physicians and health care professionals are driven by profit. Many work on salaries; many work in low-income, rural, or disadvantaged areas; many volunteer extra hours without pay; many donate services to those who cannot pay; and many are so disgusted with our current profit-oriented sickness treatment system that they are retiring early, switching fields, or cutting back their practice in order to make a reasonable income and no more. The rules and regulations, the threats of malpractice suits, and the problems with reimbursement have created an adversarial climate, and this, too, is a natural outgrowth of a profit-oriented sickness treatment system fueled by an adversarial and entrepreneurial legal system.

Within this adversarial and entrepreneurial "health care delivery system," there is one thing in increasingly short supply: caring. Here, again, there are many wonderful professionals who do care, but there is an emotional cost to this caring and that cost is chronic anger against the impersonal and mechanized system of sickness treatment of which we are a part. Unfortunately, the "system" seems so big and we view ourselves as so powerless that we often shut ourselves off from our feelings in self-defense, in order to be able to function on a daily basis. We believe that we cannot do anything to change it and therefore we stop seeing the problems. This process is so natural and so insidious that we do not realize how much we have learned not to see or feel the realities that influence our patients' lives. Hilfiker (1985) provides an eloquent account of the pressures physicians experience today that lead to this distancing effect. However, this problem applies increasingly to all professions.

Where is the caring in a sickness treatment system? Can profit-making and caring co-exist in the same system, and if so, how? What is our philosophy, as a society, about what constitutes health care? *Who* should have access to *how* much of it under *what* circumstances? How many of us really consider our body to be a machine that can be treated in isolation from the person who occupies that body? There is no more devastating experience than to be treated like a "thing," stripped of individuality, personality, and feelings (Goffman, 1961). Unfortunately, this experience of "thingness" is part of the daily life of most hospital patients (Cousins, 1979).

Now let us look at the concept of a health care system. The person is assumed to be responsible for his or her own health and professionals join in partnership with the person to provide a variety of services to restore the balance that is health. The person is assumed to have feelings and a personality; these are considered to be relevant to the assessment process; these are considered in planning and implementing any treatment process; the environment in which one lives is assumed to influence one's feelings, well-being, and health, and this, too, is considered to be a part of the evaluation and treatment process. It is assumed that there are a variety of people, professions, and interventions that will promote health and that the person has not only the right to select among these but even an inner wisdom that can be used to make such a selection. In this regard, it is considered a responsibility of all health professionals to educate the person about health and to provide the proper information so that the person can make an educated decision regarding selection of health care services. It is assumed that healing occurs from within, and it is the role of the professionals to create the climate that encourages such healing. A core feature of such a climate is interpersonal caring, respect for one another, and *mutual* trust on the part of the person and professional. Technology and diagnostic measurements are considered as only one feature of a complex assessment process that views subjective data as equally important. And finally, in a health care system, among professionals and patients, everyone is considered to be first-class colleagues; in the sickness treatment system, anyone who is not a physician is essentially a second-class citizen.

AGING AND DISABILITY

Aging is not a sickness. Rather, aging is literally the process of living, from birth to death, and this pattern of aging varies in rate and form in all of us. Chances are that if you survive a major physical disability for 20 years or more, you will experience a variety of situations comparable to those in a "nondis-abled" population, plus a few difficulties associated with the circumstances of your disability. In all people in the later years, the P,O,E balance is relevant in diagnosing and treating difficulties, but in persons with major physical disabilities this balance is often increasingly tenuous with advancing age. Consequently, it is for this reason that a sickness treatment system is the worst of all possible worlds for older people. With younger individuals, you can often get away by ignoring the psychosocial (P) and environmental (E) issues, but not with older people, and particularly, not if they have a preexisting disability.

The next several chapters review what we know and do not know about the process of aging with a physical disability. These chapters are arbitrarily categorized according to psychosocial, organic, and environmental variables, but such a separation is artificial as should be clear from the foregoing discussion. The focus is on physical disability in this particular book, but the concepts of psychosocial, biological–organic, and environmental (P,O,E) influences are relevant to "nondisabled" aging persons and persons with cognitive, emotional, or developmental disabilities. Spinal injury and polio will be the major disabilities discussed because the literature that exists deals primarily with these categories of physical dysfunction.

Actually, there has been very little published on the topic of aging with a physical disability per se, and, therefore, this book looks at literature which indirectly includes references to age in an attempt to sketch out the issues that are relevant for future study. It is a basic premise of this document that aging is just a continuation of the process of adjusting to a physical disability, and, therefore, the reader is urged to read, *Spinal Cord Injuries: The Psychological, Social, and Vocational Adjustment* (Trieschmann, 1980, out of print; 2nd edition, 1987, New York, Demos Publications), since this vast amount of literature is not reviewed herein. Specifically, we discuss the literature that looks at long-term issues of living with a disability, i.e., duration of disability of 20 years or more in persons 40 years of age or older.

4

Aging Bodies with Disabilities

INTRODUCTION

Aging is synonymous with the process of living, and each individual, disabled or "nondisabled," will display a different "pattern of aging" that is the interactive result of lifestyle (P), genetic factors (O), and socioeconomic status (E). In this chapter, we try to identify what we know and do not know about the biological–organic (O) aspects of the aging process. As we consider the issues of aging in those with physical disabilities, it is a bit unsettling to realize that the phenomenon of aging has not been clearly defined within the "nondisabled" population. Most gerontologists no longer consider it to be a single biological event but view it as a phenomenon with a multitude of manifestations that cannot be attributed to a single process. Blumenthal (1983) reports that rather than a single gene event, it is estimated that between 200 and 2,000 genes may be involved. Furthermore, the addition of lifestyle (psychosocial) risk factors plus environmental influences adds to the multiplicity of views within the field of gerontology. "It seems remarkable that despite the marked advances in biology and medicine over the last 50 years, or so, the spectrum of views regarding the aging-disease relationship remains about the same as it was over a century ago" (Blumenthal, 1983, p. xi). Thus, it is within this context that we add a new parameter to the discussion: Do many decades of living with a physical disability alter the aging process from what it would have been if the person did not have a physical impairment?

This seemingly simple question is itself extraordinarily complex, because, if the answer is yes, what is the nature of this alteration? (See Fig. 4-1.) If we consider aging to be a function of psychosocial, biological–organic, and environmental influences (P,O,E) in everyone, whether "nondisabled" or disabled, what is the impact of the physical disability? Does the presence of a physical disability accelerate the rate of aging and/or alter the format, the manifestations of the aging process? Obviously, this dichotomy is an artificial distinction within a systems concept and useful for discussion purposes only. If the *rate of aging*

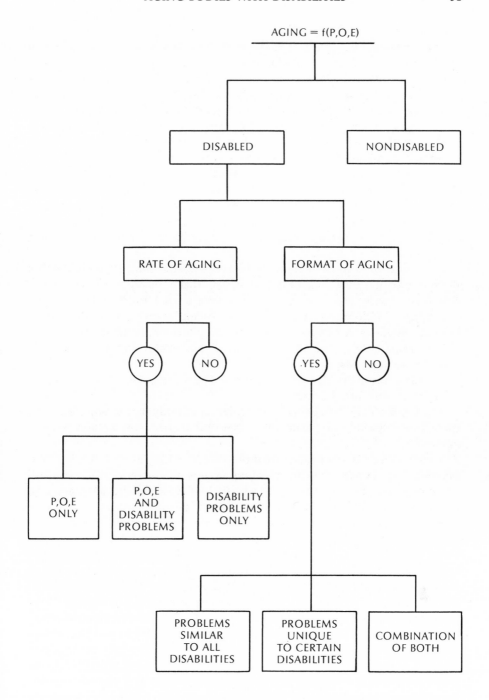

Fig. 4-1

changes (accelerates) as the result of living with a disability over several decades the question becomes: What is accelerated, the person's individualized (P,O,E) pattern and/or a constellation of dysfunctions associated with life as a disabled person? If the *format of aging* changes as a result of the disability, is it a generalized syndrome that cuts across most disabilities and/or are there specific patterns or problems associated with certain disabilities? Is the aging rate and format different for those who acquired the disability in early adult years in contrast to those who acquired it in their later years? Consequently, age of onset and duration of the disability are essential factors to be studied.

It is interesting to note that a review of the literature revealed only one article that specifically discusses the issue of patterns of aging in persons with spinal injury. Ohry et al. (1983) speculate, *but present no data to substantiate their speculations*, that persons with chronic spinal injury are subject to premature aging. Based on clinical observations at their rehabilitation center, they hypothesize the following:

1. Chronic SCIs show decreased resistance to infection. They believe that there is a greater incidence of infections and that SCIs are more resistant to antibiotic therapy as a result of long exposure to such medications.

2. Chronic SCIs may develop episodes of "silent" sepis (as seen in the elderly) often characterized by hypothermia, leukopenia, or psychiatric symptoms.

3. Chronic SCIs prematurely develop hypertension and arteriosclerotic cardiovascular disease.

4. SCIs develop bladder, prostate, and large-bowel cancers more frequently than the nonparalyzed population.

5. SCIs often exhibit changes in regulation of body temperature, stasis of body fluids, obesity, and mastopathy (males) that are similar to those in aged persons.

In sum, these authors propose that physiological functions decline at an exponential rate in persons with spinal injury, which thus reduces the physical and emotional strength available to withstand disease, fatigue, and handicap.

Any person with a spinal injury who reads the above report would have cause for great concern, and, therefore, it is important to realize that there are many persons with long-term spinal injury who have *not* exhibited these symptoms. In fact, the sample interviewed for this book on aging turned out to be remarkably healthy. It is possible, however, that this present sample was as biased as the one that Ohry et al. observed, since they describe people who were hospitalized for the very problems that they report. How representative were these persons to the total population of SCIs? What was their definition of chronic? One year post-injury, five years, 20 years? What was their definition of premature aging? At what point does a medical problem become premature? This assumes that we know the base rate of the medical problem in the population of SCIs and in the "nondisabled" population, and that this base rate information is available for age-related subgroups of each of these populations. [Base rates are the average frequency of occurrence of an event in a population.

For example, the base rate of arthritis in those aged 45–64 is 246 per 1,000 persons and 464 per 1,000 in those aged 65 and over (*Aging America: Trends and Projections,* 1984).] Consequently, this article must be viewed with great caution, rather than great alarm, and only a careful study of the population of persons with SCI *by decade in which they received their injuries* will help to elucidate some of these issues.

Unfortunately, we have *no data* in currently available research to provide definitive answers to these questions because most of the studies have not been addressed to these questions, and major methodological flaws obscure the findings in the research that has been conducted on survival of persons with SCI. However, we will look at some of these studies on survival and longevity in SCI in order to understand the nature of the methodological difficulties and problems in obtaining representative samples of persons with SCI.

LONGEVITY AND MORTALITY AFTER SPINAL CORD INJURY

Munro (1954) reports data on a group of civilian SCIs (N = 445) who were seen for treatment between 1930 and 1953. The length of the follow-up varied from hours to 20 years (a methodological problem), and data were obtained from a questionnaire but not everyone answered all questions (a biasing factor). The overall death rate was 34%, quite different from the estimated 80–90% acute mortality rate among those injured in World War I (Carroll, 1970). However, segmenting this sample into decade of onset revealed a mortality rate of 47% for those injured between 1930 and 1940 and a 20% mortality rate for those injured between 1950 and 1953. This is a good example of what happens when one averages noncomparable groups. The greatest sources of complications in those followed 18 months or more were pressure sores, bladder infections, and genitourinary tract calculi (bladder and kidney stones) associated with infections. Based on his data, Munro states, "It seems reasonable to conclude, therefore, that with proper care and rehabilitation a patient's life expectancy is not materially altered as a result of any injury of the spinal cord and cauda equina provided he has survived for at least eighteen months" (Munro, 1954, p. 13).

Dietrick and Russi (1958) describe the autopsy records of 55 persons with spinal injury at a VA hospital; as a result, their sample consists of only those who died in their hospital between 1946 and 1955 and includes both traumatic (75%) and nontraumatic cases. Average age at death was 37.7 years. In their group, average length of life after injury for those dying before 1950 was 34.9 months, whereas, after 1950, the average length of life was 71.3 months. Primary pathological diagnoses at death were: renal disease (infections and obstructions, including renal amyloidosis), 20.3%; liver disease (cirrhosis, hepatitis, and hepatic amyloidosis), 14.5%; acute abdominal catastrophe (with and without peritonitis), 10.9%; generalized infection, 9.1%; trauma, 9.1%; and cardiovascular, 7.3%. In addition to the primary diagnosis, 90% had some genitourinary disease, usually widespread; 69% had decubitus ulcers; generalized secondary amyloidosis was found in 24% and liver disease in 57%. It is quite obvious that this report documents the range of organic problems which a rather unhealthy subgroup of the spinal injury population experienced at that time, but what percentage of the total SCI population this represents cannot be estimated. In the 1940s and 1950s, the rehabilitation field was preoccupied with helping people survive, increasing their longevity, and identifying the reasons for early death. Thus, in order to justify the cost of and development of the field of rehabilitation, many of these early studies were content to ask, "How long do they live?"

Returning to the civilian world, Freed et at. (1966) report the survival experience of 243 persons with traumatic SCI who were covered by Worker's Compensation. Records of all persons from 1941 to 1964 were reviewed, and the sample included 166 paraplegics and 77 quadriplegics. Reported mortality rate was 22% (N = 54). Higher age at onset was associated with a higher death rate (a fact that has remained true today). Disorders of the genitourinary tract accounted for 25.9% of the deaths, equally divided between sepsis (infection) and renal failure. Disorders of the cardiovascular system accounted for 37% of the deaths. Infections other than urinary tract constituted 9.2% of the group and malignancy 7.4%. Of these 54 deaths, 10 occurred within two months of injury and 44 in the months and years thereafter. In the latter groups average survival time was 7.3 years with an average age of 37 years.

Nyquist and Bors (1967) report on 2,011 SCIs treated at the Long Beach VA (originally called the Birmingham VA in Van Nuys, California) between 1946 and 1965. This sample includes traumatic and nontraumatic onset, new injuries and old injuries. Of the traumatic injuries (N = 1,851), 258 or 14% were dead by 1965. Of the original group of 180 injured during World War II, 132 or 73% had survived for over 20 years, a very promising figure. Of those who survived, most were less than age 40 at onset. Of the total 258 deaths in those with traumatic injuries, renal failure accounted for 33% and was most likely to occur in the second five-year period following injury (8%). Thus, these authors state that, if a person survives 15 years without serious renal complications, the probability of death from renal failure declines. For example, in those with a duration of injury of 16–20 years, 3% died of renal failure; with a duration of 21+ years, 1% died of renal problems.

Secondary amyloidosis (protein-like deposits in tissues as the result of multiple infections) was diagnosed as cause of death in 9.6%; respiratory problems, 6.9% (73% were quadriplegic); suicide, self-neglect, and questionable accidents, 12%; vascular problems, 19%; neoplasm, 6.2%. They conclude that later age of onset and higher level of lesion are associated with shorter longevity, not only as a result of decline of life expectancy in general but because of reduced body resistance, insufficient to cope with the sequelae of injury (such as bladder and bowel dysfunction, loss of sensation, loss of mobility).

It is interesting to compare these data with the less promising data presented by Hackler (1977) 10 years later. He describes a prospective study of 270 SCIs from World War II (25 years after injury) and the Korean War (20 years) in which the mortality rates were 63 and 26%, respectively, with a combined mortality rate of 49%. This is another example of averaging disparate groups and arriving at a figure that describes neither because it masks massive group differences. The lack of comparability of the groups involves current age, duration of injury, and era of acute medical management as a minimum, all factors that influence outcome. This methodological error is present in almost all survival and longevity studies. Hackler finds renal disease to be the leading cause of death (43%) and does not find the dramatic decline in deaths from renal disease with increasing duration of disability that Nyquist and Bors found. However, he does report an increase in deaths from vascular causes with increasing duration of injury (and age, obviously). Vascular deaths account for 27% of his deaths. He also studied 175 living SCI persons, anyone who was admitted to the hospital within the last two years before the study and who had a duration of injury of at least 20 years. (This is a biased sample, by definition an unhealthy one, because it excludes those not requiring hospital admission. Thus, these figures probably overestimate the incidence of medical problems.) Fifty-nine percent had normal kidneys and another 23% had evidence of chronic pyelonephritis. Normal kidney function was found in 66% of the catheter-free group and 50% of those with Foley catheters. Hypertension was noted (diastolic pressure greater than 90) in 21% of the living patients (average age of 49 years). Of the blacks in the living group, 37% had hypertension; for whites, it was 16%. Interestingly, they report an industrial study on non-SCI men showing a prevalence rate for hypertension of 26% for whites and 36% for blacks in the 45–54 age range. Thus, in this study, in which there is a higher probability of overestimating the incidence of medical problems than actually exist in the SCI population, the hypertension incidence seems to be normal. The researcher must be commended for giving the base rates for hypertension in the general population, one of the few examples of providing base-rate information in the SCI literature.

Le and Price (1982) describe causes of death in a sample of 417 persons with SCI observed at their center between 1963 and 1976. Duration of lesion at first examination ranged from two months to 10 years; age at first examination varied from 14 to 81 years. They report that 28 persons died from the following causes:

Cause	Average duration (years)	Average age (years)
Cardiovascular (N = 7; 25%)	15	54
Respiratory (N = 6; 21%)	7	45
Suicide (N = 6; 21%)	4.3	28.5
Urinary tract (N = 4; 14%)	15	30
Miscellaneous (N = 5; 18%)	8.2	47

Unfortunately, the ages of the individuals and durations of disability vary tremendously, and the number of cases is so small that these variables preclude any reliable interpretation of these results. This does not deter these researchers, however, who concluded that average longevity of spinal-injured persons in their part of the United States is nine years with cardiovascular dysfunction as the leading cause of death! This is a most unwarranted conclusion.

Frisbie and Kache (1983) report survival and cause of death of 923 patients seen at some time over a nine-year period at the West Roxbury, Massachusetts, VA. However, they include traumatic and nontraumatic injuries in their sample and have wide variations in duration of paralysis and age at death associated with the various causes of death. Respiratory causes are first (31%); however, 76% of these are quadriplegics. Vascular system is second (28%) with an equal distribution by level of injury; gastrointestinal system, third (14%) with one-third quadriplegic; and urinary system, fourth (12%) with two-thirds quadriplegic. Cancer, rather than being a separate category, is included in the above categories. Thus, each researcher has chosen to define the categories of mortality-related events differently, which distorts the comparison of results across studies. Furthermore, there is a large standard deviation both for age at death and duration of injury, suggesting tremendous variability within these groups, which also precludes any reliable conclusions.

Nuseibeh and Burr (1982) describe the survival time of persons with paraplegia (traumatic and nontraumatic), admitted to their center between 1944 and 1969, following the occurrence of a stone in the urinary tract. Not only does the sample include nontraumatic diagnoses, but the date of onset ranges from 1913 to 1969, and the delay between injury to admission was from hours to 50 years. The group comprised 4,688 persons of whom 1,025 had died. For those with calculi, the average survival times were long, varying from 18 years for a bladder stone at age 25 to 12 years for bilateral kidney stone at the same age.

Geisler et al. (1977) attempted to contact the 1,501 persons with traumatic SCI who had been treated at Lyndhurst Lodge in Toronto between 1945 and 1973. However, they were able to obtain data on only 98.5% of the 1,501 persons, which is a sample of 1,478. Nevertheless, all of the data given in this article are based on N = 1,501. Unfortunately, this is a violation of the most basic principles of research methodology. To be included, the person had to survive the first acute hospital admission and be transferred to Lyndhurst for rehabilitation; thus, we have excluded all early deaths. None had participated in an intermittent catheterization program. Forty-nine were still hospitalized at Lyndhurst for first rehabilitation; thus, again the diversity in age and duration of disability in this sample is tremendous. Using their number of 1,501, 428 or 26% were known to be dead; this would be 29% of the N = 1,478. Renal failure accounted for 30.8%; cardiovascular, 20.4%; respiratory, 12.2%; neoplasm, 9.8%; cerebrovascular accident, 6.8%; pressure sores, 4.4%; suicide, 4.2%. Women totaled

13.2% of the 1,501 persons in the sample but accounted for only 10.8% of the deaths. Cause or duration by gender are not presented. They report that there are increased deaths in the SCI group in comparison to "nondisabled" Canadians as a result of cardiovascular disease, respiratory problems, suicide, and neoplasm in diverse sites.

In 1983, Geisler et al. updated their data to include the period from 1973 to 1980; thus, the total period is 1945–1980. During this period, they saw a total of 1,938 persons. Of this group, 428 had died by 1973, leaving 1,510 patients. (This is discrepant from the 1,501 figure reported in their 1977 article.) Of the 1,510, 1,478 were located in 1980, and there had been 194 deaths since 1973. (This gets very confusing.) They compare cause of death in 1973 and 1980 and find that, in the latter years, "other" ranks first as cause of death (26.9%). This category includes homicide, accidents, diabetes, incarcerated ventral hernia, perforated bowel, infection of bone and decubiti, septicemia, gastrointestinal hernia, bowel necrosis, and gangrene of the gallbladder. Second most frequent cause of death was cardiovascular (19.6%); renal, 15.3%, was third; respiratory, 13.9%, fourth; and neoplasm, 9.8%, fifth. Again we have only group averages and no information on level of injury, age at death, and duration of disability associated with these causes. They interpret their data to indicate that the SCI population is not at increased risk for the development of cancer.

Prior to and during World War II, a large majority of persons with traumatic spinal injury died within a month or two of genitourinary, respiratory, or infectious complications. The introduction of sulfanilamides, antibiotics, and new techniques of urinary management changed the outlook for survival, and in the late 1940s there was, for the first time, a sizable population of persons living with spinal injury. The questions repeatedly asked were, "How long will they live?" "From what will they die?" "Does it pay to provide rehabilitation?" These three questions have been the catalyst for each of the studies reviewed, but the researchers, unfortunately, overlooked the complexity of these questions and have not controlled for the variety of variables that influence the answer to these questions. Furthermore, are these really the questions that are most relevant today in the late 1980s? Nevertheless, let us explore some of the methodological issues that need to be considered in order to determine longevity and mortality in all aging and disability research.

METHODOLOGICAL ISSUES IN AGING AND DISABILITY RESEARCH

There are numerous methodological difficulties evident in all of the medical research on SCI reviewed for this book. These problems weaken or even negate the conclusions proposed by the researchers. The problems fall broadly into two categories: obtaining a representative sample and research procedures.

Sampling Problems

Traumatic Versus Nontraumatic Onset

It is essential that research on biological–organic (O) functioning differentiate between those with paraplegia and quadriplegia as a result of traumatic spinal cord injury in contrast to onset from nontraumatic causes (polio, multiple sclerosis, cancer, vascular disorders) because the *format* of the "aging" process *may be* different, whereas the format of the physical disability itself *is* quite different. For example, those with polio usually have unimpaired sensation and unimpaired bladder and bowel function. Furthermore, the "format of aging" may be quite different for polio on some dimensions than for traumatic SCI, as will be discussed below. Those with multiple sclerosis may, indeed, be functionally categorized as paraplegic or quadriplegic, but the varying constellation of symptoms associated with demyelinating disease introduces a tremendous variability to the format of the disability and the aging process. Not only are there differences across individuals, but there can be a variability of symptoms within the same individual over time. They may, or may not, have impaired sensation and bladder-bowel control. Consequently, studies reporting high or low incidence of death from renal problems or complications from pressure sores cannot be properly interpreted unless traumatic and nontraumatic onset are considered to be separate categories.

Age at Onset

There is evidence that onset of spinal injury in older persons is associated with a higher mortality rate in the acute phase than for younger persons (Young et al., 1982). Nyquist and Bors (1967) report that overall longevity of those acquiring SCI in the older years will be shorter than for younger individuals. Thus, it does not make sense to report average longevity in a sample when these diverse groups have been combined. Otherwise, this will produce a distorted result, such as noted in the Le and Price study.

Duration of Disability

All of the studies have combined persons with varying lengths of disability when reporting cause of death. However, there is strong reason to believe that the cause of death may be different for those who die in the first 10 years after onset in comparison to those who pass away 40 years after living with the disability. Nyquist and Bors (1967) do segment their sample into duration of disability associated with renal deaths and find a declining incidence over a 20-year period. Therefore, it is possible that if a person survives the first 10 years, the chances for a normal life are good. But with all of the studies published on cause of death, none of them look at duration of disability as an independent variable. In fact, some of the studies have included in their data base those who have not yet been discharged from their initial rehabilitation hospitalization.

Age at Death or at the Time of the Study

Not only is duration of disability important but current age is very relevant when describing current biological–organic (O) function or cause of death. Both of these matters are correlated with age. Most studies lump all ages together and report cause of death for the total group. Le and Price (1982), a frequently cited study on cause of death in SCI, report cardiovascular problems as foremost and urinary tract dysfunction as fourth in cause of mortality. Yet, the average age at death for the cardiovascular group is 54 and the average age of the urinary group is 29.75. Geisler et al. have published four studies on cause of death, each study adding newly injured people (and presumably younger from what we know of the demographics of spinal injury) in an attempt to increase the total sample size. They do use life table analyses to report the increased rate of death in those with SCI in comparison to a nondisabled population, but cause of death is not reported by age and duration of disability. This leads to results that are difficult to interpret with any confidence regarding the process of aging with a disability. For example, they compare cause of death prior to 1973 with cause of death during the interval from 1973 to 1980 (Geisler et al., 1983, p. 369).

Cause of death	<1973	1973–80
Renal	30.8%	15.3%
Cardiovascular	20.4	19.6
Respiratory	12.2	13.9
Neoplastic	9.8	9.8
Cerebrovascular	6.8	4.6
Suicide	4.2	10.8
Liver/alcohol	1.2	4.1
Other	15.6	26.9

Why is there the difference in incidence of renal deaths? Other, suicide, and renal have strikingly different mortality rates, but the authors do not discuss this, unfortunately. One would predict that the median and modal age of the total sample is getting younger with each succeeding study they have published, but the impact of age is unreported.

Era of Acute Management of Disability

The circumstances of treatment (both medically and psychosocially) of newly disabled persons are vastly different today than they were 40 years ago, and this may influence the data on cause of death. Persons injured in the 1940s and earlier had many more bladder problems and infections than the current group, which heightened the probability of irreversible genitourinary damage, amyloidosis (resulting from repeated infections), and decreasing effectiveness of antibiotics from long-term use. One could speculate that only the hardiest have survived 30, 40, and 50 years given the state of medical management in those days in addition to the grim psychosocial situation most disabled persons faced. Even when the message of imminent death was no longer communicated, most people had to fight a society that considered them to be deviant. Today, not only are the circumstances of acute management and rehabilitation extraordinarily improved, but the climate for entry into normal life is much more accepting. Thus, those injured in the 1930s–40s, 1950s–60s, and 1970s–80s may be quite different in health and cause of death. *Era of early management is correlated with duration of disability but is not synonymous with it, and, therefore, this may be one of the most important variables to be studied.*

Level and Completeness of Injury

Many of the studies report *number* of deaths by level and completeness but cause of death does not include these data. Nyquist and Bors (1967) report these data, plus duration of disability, for renal deaths, but this is the only example of such an analysis. Frisbie and Kache (1983) report level of injury but not completeness. When we look at the role of respiratory complications, for example, level of injury is important as are age and duration of disability, since persons with quadriplegia are more vulnerable to such problems. Death rate is higher, the higher the level of injury, but is cause of death the same over the decades? Is the format and rate of aging different in paraplegia and quadriplegia? In my interview sample, those with quadriplegia reported fewer arthritic and musculoskeletal problems than those with paraplegia but more problems with autonomic dysreflexia (sudden rise in blood pressure). Paraplegics, however, reported more upper extremity difficulties, perhaps because of greater physical mobility. Thus, one wonders if those with quadriplegia who do survive for 20 or more years may have fewer or different problems because they were capable of less physical independence.

Veteran Versus Civilian Sample

Those with a service-connected physical disability have first priority for medical care at the VA hospitals, need incur no personal medical expense, and have the financial cushion of the VA disability compensation. These are three powerful environmental (E) variables that can have a major impact on health status. As a result, are there differences in health status between service-connected and nonservice-connected disabled veterans? A study of this question would be an interesting investigation of the role of environmental resources on health as long as all of the above variables were controlled. Civilians have a different access to and costs associated with medical management depending on their source of medical coverage. Consequently, many of them may not have had the same opportunity to receive proper medical care for certain early, interim, or aging problems. Quite simply, ability to pay determines access to proper medical management in a majority of cases. Moreover, this factor should be considered in comparing outcome statistics in veteran and civilian groups.

Gender

Nationally, males account for approximately 80% of our new spinal cord injuries today. Few studies include females, and, even when women are in the group, analysis of the data by gender has been ignored. Geisler et al. (1977) have reported the incidence of death but not cause by gender. Women accounted for 13% of the sample but only 10% of the deaths. Why? Do women tend to die of different causes, at different ages, at different durations of disability than their male counterparts? This is a very interesting question.

Research Procedures

Representativeness of the Sample

In order to be able to draw conclusions about the variables examined in the study, we need to determine what other variables may confound the results and try to hold these constant. The above section on sampling outlined many of the variables that can influence the results of spinal injury. Furthermore, in order to generalize the results obtained on the study sample to a larger group of persons with spinal injury, we need to insure that the study sample is as representative of the larger group as possible. This is partly accomplished by defining the study sample by age, level and completeness of injury, duration, etc., but also by insuring that our procedures for selecting people into the study do not inadvertently bias the results.

Many of the studies reviewed in this book on aging have biased samples. Studies of survival that have a varying interval between onset of injury and entry into the study population will be biased in favor of higher survival rates because the highest mortality is within the first two weeks after onset. Studies of incidence of death or of organic dysfunction in SCI that use, as a sample, only those seeking treatment at a hospital will be biased toward a higher incidence because those who are problem-free are automatically excluded. Typical strategies to ensure representativeness include the use of control groups, prospective studies, or random samples of those not seeking treatment for anything. The latter approach has great merit.

In order to determine incidence figures for any defined organic condition, it is important to seek a random sample of persons who are not seeking medical treatment for anything. Some studies use persons hospitalized for other conditions as their sample, yet such persons are, by definition, in a state of psychological, biological–organic, environmental (P,O,E) imbalance and more likely to have health problems. If a researcher assumes that the body is a machine that can be isolated into its component parts, i.e., that only biological–organic (O) variables are relevant, a sample hospitalized for other conditions will satisfy his or her requirements for random selection. However, researchers who

view the human as a P,O,E system and believe that no body part is truly isolated from the others will want to select a sample from the SCI population at
large. Thus, it is all a matter of philosophy after all.

Control Groups

In order to study the rate and format of aging, it will be necessary to use control groups. Geisler et al. (1983) must be commended for using mortality rates
of "nondisabled" Canadians in an effort to determine comparative mortality,
and Hackler (1977) refers to incidence of hypertension in the "nondisabled"
male population of comparable age and race. Thus, we need to assess the
incidence of dysfunctions in disabled and "nondisabled" individuals and
across different groups of disabilities in an attempt to bring order to the data. If
the sample to be studied is composed of those seeking treatment, a control
group of those not seeking treatment, matched on all of the relevant variables,
must be obtained for the results to have any meaning.

Prospective Versus Retrospective Studies

The easiest type of research comes from getting a brilliant idea and deciding
to study it in a captive population, i.e., anyone who has crossed your doorstep
and left evidence of passage (a medical record). Unfortunately, what seems
easy on the surface is devilishly difficult if one intends to conduct a carefully
controlled study. The medical record, as a source of research data, is seriously
flawed because of inaccuracies and incompleteness of data entries. Furthermore, that sample is usually unrepresentative of the total population, and,
therefore, a control group is necessary but difficult, if not impossible, to obtain.
Consequently, the investigator is forced to use only those cases on which data
are available, which further biases the results in unknown ways. Such are the
pitfalls of retrospective research.

Prospective research may seem more difficult on the surface, and it certainly
involves a greater investment of time, but the results will be more valid in the
long run. In this case, a study is designed to collect data in the future that will
hopefully answer the questions asked. Therefore, there is a greater opportunity to select an unbiased sample and control for confounding variables.

Definition of Cause of Death or Dysfunction

It is impossible to compare the causes of death across the studies reviewed in
this book for all of the above-mentioned reasons but also because different investigators have defined causes of death differently. In some studies, neo-
plasms are a separate category; in others, carcinoma is included under the body
system involved. Cardiovascular includes cerebrovascular events in some
studies; in others, they are separate. Pulmonary embolism is categorized either
as a vascular or pulmonary event, depending on the investigator. Thus, the
percentages of cardiovascular, pulmonary, cancer, and renal deaths have no

generalizable meaning, and individual studies cannot be compared with each other. As a result, after all of these studies, we really do not know the cause of death in people with long-term disability.

Group Averages

Most of the studies of longevity and mortality seem to have *deified the group average*. All people with SCI of different durations, ages, levels and completeness of injury, and era of early management are grouped together and average survival time is presented! In 1954, Munro made an eloquent case for the value and necessity of rehabilitation because people with spinal injury do live long periods of time and can lead happy and productive lives. That answer has been given over and over and over, but the question never seems to change. Consequently, we still have articles that ask how long do they live and distorted group averages of nine years are given in answer. However, a significant group of persons have been living with their disabilities for 30, 40, and 50 years, and they want answers to a very different set of questions.

Causes of Death Related and Unrelated to Injury

Some authors in the above studies have tried to categorize some causes of death (renal, for example) as related to injury and others as unrelated (cardiovascular). However, this distinction is exceedingly tenuous if you view the human body as a psychosocial, biological–organic, environmental (P,O,E) system. When one has lived with a disability for many years, there is actually no cause of death that is isolated from the fact that the person has had a major physical impairment. A consistent report from my informants is a decline in energy that has significantly influenced their level of function. How can one isolate this decline in energy from susceptibility to organ and joint dysfunctions or infections? If there is a decline in energy that occurs earlier than in the "nondisabled" population of similar age, does this trigger genetic predispositions to cardiac or neoplastic problems? Consequently, it is a waste of time to make arbitrary distinctions between disability-related and disability-unrelated causes of death because there are many more important questions that need answering.

Data Collection Methodology

In many of the studies reviewed here, it is not clear how the researchers acquired their information that determined outcome or results of the study. Was it by telephone interview, mailed questionnaire, personal interview, medical exam, laboratory procedures? Was the methodology standardized so that each person was evaluated in the same manner? Were the same data available on all persons or were there gaps in the data on certain persons? What caused these gaps in data? Do these gaps in themselves bias the results in a positive or negative direction?

Size of the Sample for Low-Incidence Problems

When studying a problem that has a low frequency of occurrence in a population, any sample selected to assess the incidence of this problem must not only be representative of the entire population but must be large enough to obtain fairly accurate estimates that can be generalized to that population. The issue of bladder cancer is a perfect example of this methodological problem. Bladder cancer is a low-incidence disorder in the spinal-injured population, it would seem, and, therefore, samples must be sufficiently large to avoid the major discrepancies in incidence, as has been noted in some studies described below.

Descriptive Statistics and Tests of Statistical Significance

All of the studies reviewed herein rely on descriptive statistics, i.e., frequency, average, percentage, to report the results of the research. However, few use statistical tests to determine if the difference in incidence of problems occurred through chance or as a result of valid and reliable differences in the samples studied. For example, Le and Price (1982) report the leading cause of death as cardiovascular conditions based on seven cases, whereas respiratory conditions accounted for six deaths, suicide for six deaths, urinary tract problems for four deaths, and miscellaneous for five deaths. Just by eyeballing these data, it is obvious that these differences are not statistically significant, and, therefore, no conclusions can be drawn on cause of death from this study without even considering the diversity of age and duration of disability discussed previously.

This review of the major methodological flaws in most of the research into longevity and mortality in SCI reveals that the investigators have seriously underestimated the difficulty and complexity of the issues associated with good-quality research. On the one hand, this is a methodological problem that can be fairly easily remedied by taking a course in research design and procedure or by including expert researchers on the investigative team. On the other hand, it is a philosophical problem; it is a reflection of the operation of the sickness treatment model within medical rehabilitation. Implicit in these studies is the concept that only biological–organic (O) issues are relevant and that the body is a mechanism that can be fragmented into parts for study. It is important to note that the view of the human as a psychosocial, biological–organic, environmental (P,O,E) system does not imply that quantifiable and controlled research is impossible. Rather, it implies that there are a multitude of variables that can influence the one under study. These must be recognized and attempts made to "control" their impact on the research result. Thus, when the rest of the medical community dismisses rehabilitation research as not hard, or even good, science, unfortunately the quality of much of this research provides ample evidence to substantiate this criticism.

HEALTH PROBLEMS ASSOCIATED WITH LONG-TERM SPINAL CORD INJURY

As noted above, only Ohry et al. (1983) have directly addressed the issue of the type of organic dysfunctions that persons with long-term SCI might experience, but they provide no data to back up their hypotheses. We have reviewed a selection of studies on longevity and mortality to elucidate this issue of aging and disability but find it impossible to draw any firm conclusions because of major methodological flaws in these studies. In a further attempt to identify what we know and do not know about aging and spinal cord injury, let us look at research on renal disease, cardiovascular problems, and other organic dysfunctions that may occur in the lives of those with long-term SCI.

Renal Disorders

Historically, most of the deaths in persons with spinal cord injury were associated with renal dysfunction, and such deaths occurred within several years of injury. However, the introduction of sulfanilamides, antibiotics, and greater knowledge about bladder management have altered this pattern so that fewer people die early from kidney dysfunction, and those who survive to the later years have the opportunity to acquire other disorders that account for the deaths in the "nondisabled" population.

Nyquist and Bors (1967) found that renal failure accounted for 32.9% of the 258 deaths in their sample, which was 5% of the 1,851 persons with traumatic SCI in their sample. Remembering that this sample was treated between 1946 and 1965, these figures include a large number of persons injured in the earlier era of SCI management. They note a varying percentage of mortality in this group by duration (in years) of disability:

1–5	6–10	11–15	16–20	21+
5%	8%	5%	3%	1%

Thus, they state that if a person survives 15 years without serious renal complications, the probability of death from renal failure declines.

Studying a World War II and Korean War group of SCI (again early era of management), Hackler (1977) noted 43% deaths from renal problems; however, with increasing years post-injury, the number of renal deaths declined slightly and the number of cardiovascular deaths increased. Renal amyloidosis was found in many of these individuals, but we cannot rely on exact figures, since post-mortem examinations were not conducted on all who died.

Those who died of urinary tract problems were younger (average age of 29.75) than those who died of many other problems in the Le and Price (1982) study, and these deaths ranked fourth as cause of death.

Thirty percent of the deaths were associated with renal failure in the sample described by Geisler et al. (1977), but we need to remember that duration of disability varied widely, as did era of early SCI management and age at onset of disability. Incidence of renal death by age group revealed that 54% of these deaths occurred prior to age 50, whereas 71% of the cardiovascular deaths occurred after age 50. In a later study (Geisler et al., 1983), these authors report that 15% of the deaths between 1973 and 1980 resulted from renal failure (other, 26.9%; cardiovascular, 19.6%; respiratory, 13.9%; suicide, 10.8%), but we do not have any knowledge of duration of disability or age of those who died in this interval.

Nuseibeh and Burr (1982) studied the survival time in paraplegics with urinary complications, but their sample includes many with nontraumatic injuries; as a result, there is considerable difference in bladder function in this group. There are other methodological flaws that make this a most unrepresentative sample; however, they note that death after diagnosis of bladder stone at age 25 occurred an average of 18 year later. But it is difficult to generalize this to other than their particular sample.

It is particularly frustrating to be unable to document precisely the role of renal dysfunction as a cause of death in traumatic spinal injury when physicians have been trumpeting the importance of the genitourinary system as a factor in long-term survival. Methods of bladder management have changed in the last 40 years, and the advent of antibiotics has reduced the frequency and virulence of bladder infections in this population. Consequently, era of acute SCI management is a critical variable in any exploration of this topic. Duration of disability is a related but separate issue, since there is suggestive evidence that major renal dysfunction will be apparent in the first 20 years after onset. The role of amyloidosis in death from renal dysfunction needs to be clarified, since it infiltrates body organs as a result of multiple infections. Is amyloidosis correlated with either era of acute SCI management or duration of disability? Does type of bladder management strategy influence the incidence of death from renal disease or are amyloidosis, multiple calculi, and repeated infection the major culprits regardless of type of bladder management? Does intermittent catheterization influence the outcome?

Now we have the advent of hemodialysis, which extends the life of those with end-stage renal disease (ESRD) by several years. Unfortunately, we do not know what percent of the SCI population reaches this stage and receives this treatment. Vaziri (1984a,b) reports 60% survival for one year and 52% for two years in a group of 40 SCI treated at the Long Beach VA. Survival rates for non-SCIs on dialysis are 80% for one year. Sepsis and other bacterial infections are the main cause of death in dialysis patients with SCI, whereas cardiovascular disease is the leading cause of mortality in those who are not spinal-injured but on dialysis.

Barton et al. (1984b) describe the renal pathology found on autopsy of 21 SCI-ESRD patients treated with maintenance hemodialysis at Long Beach between 1973 and 1979. Autopsy findings on 43 non-SCI dialysis patients who expired during the same time were also examined. The SCI group had an average age of 46 and average duration of disability of 20.7 years (range, 6–32). Duration of dialysis was 17 months (range, 1–60). The non-SCI-ESRD patients averaged an age of 54 years and were on dialysis an average of 43 months (range, 1–70).

Chronic pyelonephritis was present in 100% of the SCI cases and 27.9% of the non-SCI cases. Amyloidosis occurred in 81% of the SCIs and 4.7% of the non-SCIs. Primary cause of death in SCIs was Gram-negative sepsis (61.9%); in non-SCIs, 32.5% had an acute myocardial infarction, 16.3% had broncho-pneumonia, 16.2% had cardiomyopathy, and 11.6% had sepsis as primary cause of death. Pneumonia and cardiac conditions were low-frequency causes of death in these SCIs. Interestingly, clinical hypertension was found in only 33% of the SCIs in contrast to 88% of the non-SCI group. The authors speculate that the etiology of the ESRD was different in the two groups: chronic pyelonephritis in SCIs, general circulatory problems in non-SCIs.

This same group of SCI-ESRD patients was examined for cardiovascular pathology on autopsy (Pahl et al., 1983), but unfortunately no control group of non-SCI-ESRD is presented for comparison purposes. Thus, the results do not help us to understand the role that SCI plays. Coronary arteriosclerosis was found in 45% of the cases, yet myocardial infarction was rare. Mild cardiac amyloidosis was found in 25%. One would presume that the incidence of cardiovascular pathology would be even higher in the non-SCI-ESRD group given the findings of Barton et al. (1984b) described above.

Vaziri et al. (1982c) reported lipid abnormalities in 10 SCI-ESRD patients undergoing hemodialysis and a group of SCIs without ESRD. Since we know that there were 40–43 patients in this ESRD group studied by Vaziri at Long Beach, why were these 10 chosen? Are these a representative sample of the original group? Average age in this sample was 59, whereas average age of the total group was 46! Does the probability of finding lipid abnormality increase with age? Total serum triglycerides were higher in SCI-ESRDs (180 mg/dl) than SCI-non-ESRDs (100 mg/dl) and non-SCIs (104 mg/dl). There was no significant difference in serum cholesterol between SCI-ESRDs (152 mg/dl) and SCI-non-ESRDs (142 mg/dl), and both were lower than non-SCIs (224 mg/dl)! However, high-density lipid (HDL) cholesterol was significantly lower in SCI-ESRDs (12 mg/dl) than in SCI-non-ESRDs (31 mg/dl), and both were lower than normals (49 mg/dl). HDL cholesterol is considered to be "good," and its presence seems to lower the risk or coronary artery disease in contrast to low-density lipoprotein (LDL) cholesterol, which was not measured. It would be interesting to check lipid levels in a large group of SCIs of different ages and durations of disability and compare with non-SCIs the risk of coronary artery disease.

Hematological features of the total group of 43 SCI-ESRDs were reported by Vaziri et al. (1982a). A control group of 45 non-SCI-ESRD patients was used for comparison. SCI patients displayed a moderate to severe anemia, necessitating multiple transfusions, probably caused by chronic renal failure and chronic bacterial infections.

Ninety-eight percent of these 43 patients had active chronic urinary tract infections with multiple organisms found in 48% (Vaziri et al., 1982b). Pressure sores were present in 63% with multiple organisms in 55%. Septicemia occurred in over half of the 22 on whom autopsies were performed and was the cause of death in 11. Amyloidosis of the endocrine glands was found in 15 of the 43 patients by Barton et al. (1984*a*) and of the gastrointestinal tract in 13 patients by Meshkinpour et al. (1982). Protein calorie malnutrition was found in this group by Mirahmadi et al. (1983).

Although further research must be conducted to test these hypotheses, it is possible that death from renal failure may be partly associated with the era of acute and subacute SCI management. Amyloidosis was found pervasively in most organs of those on whom autopsies were conducted. This condition is a direct result of multiple infections: bladder, renal, pressure sores. It seems likely that those injured in the 1940s had a history of more bladder infections than those more recently injured. If these individuals, then, have repeated bouts of decubiti, the probability of amyloidosis increases. The same problem can occur today but would be less frequent in incidence, one would hypothesize. However, these are issues for future research.

There is reason to believe that death from renal failure is less likely in those with spinal injury of 20 or more years who have not had consistent genitourinary problems. It seems likely that the pattern of major bladder and kidney dysfunction establishes itself within the first five years of disability and is highly correlated with "adjustment" to disability. As a result, the psychosocial, biological–organic, environmental (P,O,E) interaction is critical in this matter as it is with most health issues, assuming that proper medical management has been available to the person.

This latter issue, however, deserves attention. My interview sample represents the "crème de la crème" in terms of adjustment to disability. These people know how to take care of their bodies, and their current longevity and good health are a testament to this. However, many complain about the inordinate amount of time it takes to get the results of a urinalysis and urine culture, particularly through some of the VA outpatient departments, when they know they have a bladder infection. By the time the results are available and medication is prescribed, the infection has raged for two to three weeks. This is not good medical management of genitourinary problems.

The incidence of renal failure associated with various techniques of bladder management has not been determined. The more recent use of intermittent catheterization in contrast to external catheter use should be evaluated with duration of disability and era of acute SCI management as controlled variables. Perhaps type of bladder management is less important than number of infections over time. Thus, it is now time for some carefully controlled research into these very important issues.

Cardiovascular Conditions

The incidence of cardiovascular conditions in the spinal injury population is not known. Some of the studies on longevity and mortality in SCI have noted that cardiovascular conditions account for a significant proportion of deaths. However, from the data available, we cannot draw any firm conclusions on this matter because of the methodological problems in these studies, but also, of equal importance, because each investigator has defined the term cardiovascular differently or does not state a definition at all.

Nyquist and Bors (1967) use the term vascular deaths to include such conditions as cardiac, cerebrovascular, pulmonary embolism, generalized arteriosclerosis, ruptured aneurysm, hemorrhage from decubitus ulcer, and bacterial endocarditis. These conditions accounted for 49 of 258 (19%) deaths or 3% of the 1,851 persons with traumatic SCI in the sample. Coronary heart disease occurred in 23 persons, which is 47% of the vascular deaths, 8.9% of all deaths, and 1.2% of all traumatic SCI. A majority of these people were in their 40s; age at injury and duration of disability are not given.

Hackler (1977) found vascular deaths (defined as myocardial infarction, cerebrovascular accident, pulmonary embolism) to occur in 32 of the 137 deaths, i.e., 27%. He notes that with increasing duration of disability, renal deaths declined very slightly in his sample and vascular deaths increased markedly. By 25 years post-injury, deaths from these two conditions were almost equal. In his retrospective study of 175 living SCIs, he found the following conditions:

Hypertension	21%
Hypertensive heart disease	10%
Myocardial infarction	6%
Arteriosclerosis	9%
Diabetes mellitus	9%
Cerebrovascular accident	3%
Chronic decubitus (deep)	39%

It is important to remember that these 175 SCIs were admitted to the hospital for treatment of unspecified conditions and were at least 20 years post-injury (average, 24.2 years). Average age was 49 years (range, 42–62). Thus, this sample is biased toward overestimating the incidence of medical problems.

Le and Price (1982) report cardiovascular problems to be the leading cause of death in their sample, but we have already noted significant methodological problems with this study. Those who died of cardiovascular problems were much older than those who died of some other causes, and their sample is not representative of the SCI population on a variety of dimensions. Included in their definition are dissecting aneurysm, myocardial infarction, stroke, and orthostatic hypotension.

Geisler et al. (1977) report cardiovascular disease as the second leading cause of death in their sample (87 of 428 deaths). Unfortunately, they do not define what dysfunctions were included in this category. Keeping in mind that it is not clear exactly how they obtained information on cause of death (family report?), their data suggest that there are a greater number of deaths from cardiovascular conditions in the SCI group, aged 20–44, than in the "nondisabled" Canadian population of similar age in 1971. They report:

Lesion and age	Actual deaths	Expected
Incomplete lesions		
Age 20–44	8	2
Age 45–64	21	20
Complete lesions		
Age 20–44	11	2
Age 45–64	15	11

As will be noted, the deaths in the older age group are close to the norm for "nondisabled" Canadians. Deaths from cardiovascular conditions by decade of age reveals that 71% occur in those 50 or older:

Age	Deaths
10–19	0
20–29	2
30–39	9
40–49	14
50–59	16
60–69	27
70–79	10
79+	9

Thus, while there may be an earlier incidence of heart disease in a small segment of the SCI population, possibly related to family history plus the additional stress of living with a disability, the majority of cardiac conditions occur in an age group similar to the "nondisabled" population. Whether or not research on a larger and carefully selected sample will demonstrate this to be the case remains to be seen.

Blocker et al. (1983) looked at the electrocardiograms (EKGs) of 98 SCIs that had been performed as a routine part of their admission to a VA hospital. We, unfortunately, do not know the duration of disability, era of injury, or general medical condition of this sample. The most common abnormalities seen were S-T depressions and T-wave inversions. Abnormal EKGs were most frequently encountered in the 50–59 age group, but we do not know the duration of the disability. Level of SCI was unrelated to incidence of abnormal EKG. Unfortunately, we have no control group nor do we have essential demographic information on the SCI subjects, which would permit a clearer understanding of these results.

Dependent edema is a frequently reported difficulty in many paralyzed people. Not only does this increase the probability of pressure sores from tight-fitting shoes, but there is some question as to whether dependent edema may be associated with embolism formation, which can compromise cardiac and pulmonary function. This issue certainly deserves investigation along with studies on how to treat and prevent the edema problem. Does wrapping the dependent extremities reduce this problem?

Based on these studies, we can say that cardiovascular problems have complicated the lives of SCI persons as well as "nondisabled" individuals. Perhaps one of the more interesting outcomes of the rehabilitation movement is that a large group of people have lived long enough to acquire the "diseases of civilization": the epitome of success in western societies. Whether the incidence is higher in SCIs than in a comparable "nondisabled" group, we do not know, but there is suggestive evidence of earlier onset of cardiovascular problems in some SCIs. However, whether this is the result of genetic predisposition, stress, and other health (or nonhealth habits) as in the "nondisabled" population or the result of a specific combination of physiological factors associated with the SCI per se cannot be determined from these data. *Since cardiovascular problems are highly correlated with age, any study that does not control for this variable should not be published.* Duration of disability is a factor as well as gender.

There is a tremendous amount of research that could be done to examine the role of lifestyle on the incidence of cardiovascular conditions in a physically disabled population. Although less physically mobile on some dimensions, there is greater physical effort associated with daily living. How much cardiopulmonary conditioning results from repeated transfers and wheelchair propulsion? The issues of exercise, diet, and smoking would be expected to be relevant as in a "nondisabled" population. Many of my informants report feeling exhausted when the end of the day arrives. Will exercise increase one's energy level or accelerate the drain on total lifetime physiological reserves? Do those who participate actively in sports when younger have an advantage over less active persons in lowering the incidence of cardiac conditions? What is the effect of nutrition on energy and cardiac status in disabled persons? Do the high-fiber/carbohydrate and low-fat diets that have produced great physical performance in athletes and a wonderful sense of well-being help older disabled people cope with the declining energy problems? Are people willing to reduce their consumption of red meats to try this?

All research into these issues in samples of disabled persons *must* consider the base rate of cardiovascular conditions in the "nondisabled" population for comparison purposes. *Aging America: Trends and Projections* (1984) indicates that incidence of cardiovascular disease increases with advancing age:

Condition	17–44	45–64	65+
Hypertensive disease	54.2	243.7	378.6
Heart conditions	37.9	122.7	277.0

These figures represent number of cases per 1,000 persons. Consequently, there are many fascinating and valuable studies that can be conducted into this topic. Hopefully, future endeavors will be methodologically sound.

Bladder Cancer

In their study of spinal-cord-injured patients treated at the Long Beach VA from 1946 to 1965, Nyquist and Bors (1967) found that seven of their 1,851 traumatic SCIs died of bladder, renal, or urethral cancer. This constituted 2.7% of all deaths and 0.38% of this sample of 1,851 persons. While this mortality is higher than that reported for "nondisabled" men in 1961 (0.008%), it was not a large percentage of either the total deaths or total number of persons in the sample. Because five of the seven were catheter-free, the authors wondered if chronic infection was a factor in the etiology. Six died between 40 and 50 and one was 32 at death. Deaths occurred within two years of diagnosis and within 12–20 years after injury.

Hackler (1977) had a sample of 445 SCIs and found three deaths from bladder cancer, which was 2% of all deaths in his sample of World War II and Korean War veterans and 0.67% of his total sample.

Geisler et al. (1977) reported 12 deaths from bladder cancer, which is 2.8% of the 428 deaths or 0.79% of their sample of 1,510 persons with SCI. None of the sample had been maintained by intermittent catheterization, but form of bladder management was not stated. Duration of disability was not given, but age at death and completeness of injury revealed that eight of 12 deaths occurred in the 20–44 age range, whereas four occurred in the 45–64 age bracket. Ten of the 12 deaths occurred in individuals with complete lesions and two in those with partial lesions. It is interesting to note, however, that the bladder cancer constituted only 28.5% of all of the cancer deaths (42), and, thus, the authors note the diversity of sites in which cancer has been found in their sample of SCIs. Cancer accounted for 9.8% of all deaths in their sample.

In their later study, which had a total sample of 1,938 persons, Geisler et al. (1983) found the same mortality of cancer in diverse sites, again 9.8% of the total deaths; however, they compared actual and expected deaths from *all* cancers in SCIs and "nondisabled" Canadians:

Lesion	Actual deaths	Expected
Complete quadriplegia	3	1.3
Complete paraplegia	6	6.1
Partial quadriplegia	6	6.7
Partial paraplegia	4	8.7

They conclude, "The data does not now suggest that the spinal injured population are at a significantly increased risk to the development of cancer as had been earlier supposed" (Geisler et al., 1983, pp. 370–371). They do not discuss mortality from bladder cancer as a separate category, however.

Investigating the issue of bladder cancer specifically, Kaufman et al. (1977) found two patients with diffuse squamous cell carcinoma of the bladder and decided to do a prospective study of SCI persons managed with and without indwelling bladder catheters. Their subject sample consisted of 62 SCIs who had been hospitalized for other than urological problems or were seen as outpatients for yearly routine evaluation. The proportion of each is not presented. Thus, this cannot be considered to be a random sample of healthy persons with SCI. They used as a control group 12 "nondisabled" individuals hospitalized for transurethral resection of benign prostatic hypertrophy or bladder tumors. The patients were categorized by type of bladder management and the pathologist was unaware from which group the biopsy material was received.

They report an incidence of squamous cell carcinoma of the bladder in six of 62 SCIs (10%), which includes the two original cases that instigated the prospective study. Unfortunately, this is a major methodological error, which inflates the incidence figures. A prospective study should include *only* those on whom there is *no* prior information of bladder cancer status; otherwise, it is not a random sample. As a result, the actual incidence is four of 60 or 7% of their sample. Transitional cell carcinoma was also noted in most of them. The majority of these men were in their early 50s; all but one had used a catheter for bladder management. In the total sample, of those with indwelling catheters for more than 10 years, 80% had extensive squamous metaplasia; those with indwelling catheters for less than 10 years showed a 42% incidence of squamous metaplasia of the bladder. None in the control group displayed evidence of bladder cancer. The authors point to the important role that biopsy played in the diagnosis, since endoscopic exam did not reveal any abnormality beyond chronic cystitis in many cases. Thus, the issue of early detection of bladder cancers needs to be studied in order to institute early treatment and, hopefully, reduce the mortality associated with this diagnosis.

A very different finding is reported by Broecker et al. (1981) who studied prospectively 81 SCIs hospitalized at the Richmond, Virginia, VA during a one-year period. They were categorized as group 1 ($N = 50$), indwelling catheter for 10 or more years, and group 2 ($N = 31$), external catheter for 15 or more years. Biopsies were performed. No bladder cancer was found in this sample. In group 1, ages ranged from 29 to 83 years with a median of 51, and duration of injury ranged from 11 to 35 years with a median of 22; and group 2, ages 35–67 with a median of 50 years and duration of 15–34 years, median of 22 years. All showed varying degrees of chronic inflammation, but squamous metaplasia was found in only 22% of those with catheters and 8% of those without.

In a retrospective study of 1,052 new admissions to their VA since 1963, these authors found 10 cases of bladder cancer. Age range was 33–58 with a median of 48 years; duration of disability ranged from 10 to 32 years, median of 18 years. Of these 10, four had used an indwelling catheter 10–32 years, median, 20 years; two had external catheters, one for 18 and one for 12 years. One had had an ileal conduit diversion nine years after injury and three years prior to cancer diagnosis. The bladder management of the other three is not reported.

El-Masri and Fellows (1981) present the largest sample, 6,744 SCIs followed by the National Spinal Injuries Centre, Stoke Mandeville Hospital, in England.

In this group, they noted an incidence of 25 cases of bladder cancer, an incidence of 0.37% of the sample. Of these, there have been 21 deaths, 0.31% of their total sample. In comparison to the death rate from bladder cancer in "nondisabled" males in England and Wales, cord injury increased the risk by a factor of 20. Nevertheless, the actual probability of dying of bladder cancer, whether SCI or "nondisabled," is very small.

Of the 25 cases of bladder cancer, average interval between injury and diagnosis was 23 years (range, 11–42):

Age at diagnosis	No. of cases	Era of injury	No. of cases
30–39	6	<1940	3
40–49	4	1940–44	8
50–59	10	1945–49	6
60–69	5	1950–54	2
		1965–70	1

In four cases, date of injury was unknown. Seventeen had been injured prior to 1950: the authors hypothesize that the cancer may be related to bladder management techniques in the earlier days, many of the patients having suprapubic cystotomies. Incidence of upper motor neuron and lower motor neuron lesions was equal.

In evaluating these data, we can say with reasonable assurance that the incidence of bladder cancer is higher in our current population of SCIs than in the "nondisabled." However, the absolute risk of any one individual acquiring such an organic dysfunction is small. These studies have found that death from bladder cancer accounts for 0.3–3% of the *known deaths* in SCIs, yet because of methodological difficulties with most of these studies, these comments should be considered to be hypotheses for future research. In the various samples, 0.31–0.79% of the *total number* of SCIs in the sample died of bladder cancer. How representative these samples are remains to be seen. Most of these cancers have been detected in the age range of 30–50, and the duration of disability has been more than 10 years. However, there is strong suggestive evidence that era of acute SCI management may be a major variable, as noted by El-Masri and Fellows (1981). There is speculation as to whether it is type of bladder management (indwelling catheter versus external drainage) or the history of frequent and severe bladder infections in the early years that is the predisposing factor. Consequently, comparisons of incidence by *era of injury* (not necessarily the same as duration) would be exceedingly interesting. Because the incidence of bladder cancer is relatively low, large samples will have to be studied to prevent sampling errors from occurring. The error possible in small samples is obvious when comparing the study by Kaufman et al. (1977) who found an incidence of 7% and Broecker et al. (1981) who found a 0% incidence, both using hospitalized samples of less than 100 each. If era of injury is a powerful influence on the incidence of bladder cancer, then we would hope to see the incidence decline even further. Thus, if the data above are confirmed by future research, the probability of bladder cancer is even lower if one or more of the following apply: you were injured after 1950; you have had your injury for 20 of more years; you are age 53 or older. Naturally, these are hypotheses for future research.

The issue of early diagnosis deserves some consideration. Kaufman et al. (1977), who found the highest incidence, report that the cancer would have not been detected without biopsy in most of the cases. Since squamous cell cancer has a poor prognosis by the time that clinical signs are grossly evident, we need to diagnose and treat it as early as possible. However, it will also be important to evaluate the cost benefits of generalized screening using invasive techniques for a relatively low incidence, albeit deadly, disorder. Family history of cancer may be a predisposing factor, but era of acute injury seems to be our best lead at the present.

Autonomic Dysreflexia

Those persons with spinal injuries at or above T4-6 are vulnerable to autonomic dysreflexia: a sudden rise in blood pressure that could be fatal if untreated. Bladder or bowel problems may trigger an episode, and occasionally orthostatic hypotension can produce a rebound effect of sudden hypertension. Several individuals interviewed for this report noted an increasing incidence of such problems; most of these were women. They have found that most physicians and emergency rooms have no idea what the problem is, how serious it could be, or what to do about it. A review of the literature revealed no articles that report data on this problem in long-term SCI.

According to Judith C. Gilliom (1985), participant in the Long Range Planning Conference of the National Institute for Handicapped Research, investigative efforts to date have focused on newly injured persons, perhaps because they are readily accessible as inpatients. However, the older generation of SCIs has been almost totally ignored. Little is known about the typical patterns of autonomic dysfunction in individuals who have been injured for 10 years or more. Some physicians believe that this problem stabilizes over time and becomes less of a management issue. However, according to many persons with quadriplegia, this is not the case at all. Unfortunately, this problem has been considered to be a nuisance rather than a continuing impediment to a normal lifestyle. Because we have not really looked carefully at the health status of persons with long-term disability, we have no idea of the incidence of this problem nor the degree to which it disrupts normal living. Generally, interest has been directed at the basic mechanisms of autonomic dysreflexia (Frankel and Mathias, 1979) rather than at methods of prevention and treatment. Not only do we need to explore the incidence and dimensions of this problem, but we need to plan specific strategies to disseminate this information to general practitioners and emergency rooms. Many a person with high-level spinal injury has felt literally abandoned by the medical profession when they have sought help in dealing with an acute episode of autonomic dysreflexia. However, many an expert in spinal injury has tried to educate his or her fellow physicians on this topic only to be rebuffed. Attempts to introduce lectures on this topic to family practice residents at one medical school were rejected because the problem was considered to be irrelevant to the usual practice of these physicians. Thus, education of the spinal-injured person and family is an important avenue to explore. However, before we can educate, we need to elucidate.

Without a doubt, we need to survey the population of persons with SCI at T6 and above to determine the incidence and character of this disorder. Does the pattern change within an individual over time? Are the patterns of dysfunction idiosyncratic or are there general features that cut across many individuals? Does duration of disability, present age, gender, and stress influence this problem? Once we have defined the nature of the problem, we need to explore intervention strategies. What drugs or other types of treatment are effective in treating an episode already in existence and in preventing future episodes? Emphasis should be given to the unusual forms of dysreflexia triggered by other than the customary stimuli. The results of these endeavors should be disseminated to the medical and SCI community. However, in the meantime, *specific steps should be taken to prepare posters or pamphlets for distribution to all hospital emergency rooms and paramedic squads.* Publication of articles in journals of the various medical specialties *other than* rehabilitation would reach a wider variety of practitioners and help to disseminate information to those physicians not affiliated with SCI centers.

Pressure Sores

People who have survived 30–50 years with a disability are not merely lucky; rather, they are capable, resourceful, and knowledgable about their bodies. Those who were neglectful of their self-care died long ago, and, therefore, the majority of pressure sores in our long-term disability group are probably not the result of neglect or carelessness. Some of my informants report that they are more vulnerable to pressure sores now and some report no problem in this area. What accounts for this difference? One person hypothesized that the body is less efficient in its use of nutrients, which makes the skin more vulnerable to breakdown, and healing becomes a longer process. One individual reported that his life centers around his skin, and his personal schedule is determined by whether he has any red spots when he awakens in the morning. His entire ability to plan ahead has been disrupted by this issue, which is becoming very depressing to him. Nevertheless, he and his wife have worked around his disability for 40 years and they will continue to do so. One wonders what the impact of amyloidosis in multiple body organs has on the overall efficiency of body functioning. Is this a factor in the increased susceptibility to pressure sores? Is this a factor in less efficient utilization of nutrition, if, indeed, this problem exists? Is this related to era of SCI management? Does the function of the endocrine system influence pressure sore development in the later years?

Many persons with long-term disability put on excess weight, as do the rest of us "nondisabled" but aging individuals. But the weight makes mobility more difficult with the possibility of fewer weight shifts to relieve pressure on skin and the possibility of more abrasions or bruises during transfers. Also, declining energy would compound this problem. Conversely, some people lose weight with age, which may increase the number of bony prominences and exacerbate a pressure sore problem.

Swelling in dependent extremities may be an additional factor in pressure sore incidence. Thus, many of my informants have increasing trouble finding shoes that fit properly and that do not cause skin problems.

There are numerous interesting research projects to be carried out in this area, such as the incidence of pressure sores in this group. Do these increase in incidence with age? Clinically, it will be essential to differentiate this group from those with a history of pressure sores from self-neglect. There are few situations more demoralizing to a hospital staff than someone repeatedly admitted for the same problem that could be prevented. It is natural to become frustrated and even angry with the person. However, it is probable that a large percentage of our long-term disability group do not have a previous history of repeated problems resulting from self-neglect, and, thus, they should not be perceived as part of this other group. Such subtleties in attitude on the part of the staff can make a big difference in the quality of care.

Suicide

Suicide has been listed as a frequent cause of death in SCIs in our longevity and mortality studies, and, therefore, we need to consider the relevance of this concept to long-term disability.

Nyquist and Bors (1967) report that confirmed suicide occurred in 21 of their 258 deaths (8%), 1.3% of their sample of 1,851 persons seen at the Long Beach VA between 1946 and 1965. There was no difference by level of injury, but there was for age at time of suicide: 24–29 (19%), 30–39 (57%), 41–50 (14%), 50+ (10%). However, when examining the plethora of statistics in this article, Trieschmann (1980) calculated that if one included certain deaths from questionable accidents and very preventable medical complications (passive or physiological suicide), as many as 12% of the deaths could be labeled as suicide. However, age at suicide is interesting. A majority of suicides occurred when the people were in their 30s in contrast to the "nondisabled" population in which 20% were 20–39 years old, 44% were 40–59, and 36% were 60+. Thus, in "nondisabled" persons, suicide tends to occur in older age groups, whereas in spinal injury it tends to occur earlier in the course of the disability.

Hackler (1977) found that suicide occurred in five of the 137 deaths among World War II and Korean War veterans in his sample. Le and Price (1982) report that suicide accounted for six of the 28 deaths in their sample of 417 persons.

We noted earlier in this chapter that there were varying ages and durations of disability in those who died. Those who committed suicide had the shortest duration of disability (4.3 years) and the youngest age (28.5 years). Geisler et al. (1983) report that 4.2% of the deaths in their sample up to 1973 was caused by suicide, but this figure rose to 10.8% of the deaths from 1973 to 1980. Liver/alcohol was a cause of mortality of 1.2% and 4.1%, respectively, in these study periods. As we have noted previously, these researchers added all new injuries seen at their center to the total sample with each succeeding study; presumably this accounts for the increased incidence of suicide in the latter period.

Thus, essentially suicide has been a cause of death in the earlier years of life with a disability. Many people, on finding themselves paralyzed, believe that life is not worth living and some wish that they would die. This is quite normal in the early phases of the disability because the person lacks any information that life can still have rewards, satisfactions, successes, and happiness despite the disability. Initially, all that one perceives is the loss. But most people pull it together, get through the rehabilitation program, and go out and try to do the best they can. However, within 5–10 years, the person has a fairly good idea of what life with a disability will entail, and some decide to withdraw from the game. Active suicide is an option and passive suicide (self-neglect to a dramatic degree) is another way out. Most of those who live 15 years or more with a disability appear to have decided to proceed with living and tend to do so fairly well.

Suicide does not seem to be a major cause of death in many cases in the middle to later years with disability. Whether or not this continues to be the case will be interesting to note. By definition, those who make it 30, 40, and 50 years are survivors: they have deeply ingrained habits of self-care and manage their resources carefully in order to keep going. But the length of the game, particularly in those without high incomes or financial compensation for the disability, may take its toll and the "no-win" aspects may erode even the strongest. Sally, Dave, and Jack have been constantly penalized financially in addition to the physical and emotional penalties of major disability. They have shown great resilience and resourcefulness over their lifetimes, but they are tired of the battle. Sally clings to her religious beliefs of a life after death, which is a compensation for her struggle in this life. Jack, who chose to die twice prior to his 10th anniversary of disability, has decided to take no more active steps in that regard, yet almost wishes that he would not wake up in the morning. And Dave finds that his hopes for major legislative change and enlightenment have not been realized and, thus, is searching for something to believe in, some reason to continue the daily fight to live, some reason to live. Frank, Clifford, Paul, and Bill have financial advantages that cushion the impact of declining function, and they have not experienced the same degree of spiritual and philosophical crisis that the others are going through. However, that is not to say that life with a disability does not weigh heavily on them.

But what happens when a beloved spouse dies after 40–50 years of marriage and partnership? Now the disabled person will not only be compromised in physical assistance but without a major source of emotional support. Will active or passive suicide become more frequent? I would hypothesize that it will occasionally occur but not very frequently because these people chose to live a long time ago. They have exhibited resilience, fortitude, and drive, which will continue to carry them through whatever crises the future holds. They are survivors, but it is more than that. It is probable that suicide is not now and never was consistent with the essential personality structure of these individuals. It is interesting to note, however, that the spouses tend to worry whether the disabled person will give up; but my informants report that few of them do. Naturally, these become interesting hypotheses for future research.

THE RESIDUALS OF POLIO

Not only is the group with long-term SCI experiencing a decline in function long after onset of the disability, but those with polio are experiencing a constellation of symptoms that, in some cases, has drastically changed a lifestyle and raised frightening questions of progressive deterioration. The issues of rate of aging and format of the aging process are relevant here as in our discussion of spinal injury.

Halstead et al. (1985) conducted an informal survey of post-polio survivors and analyzed the data from 201 questionnaires. Since there is not a well-defined network of post-polio individuals, the questionnaire was distributed to anyone known to have polio in several communities. As a result, the authors admit that they have no control over the representativeness of the sample and suspect that those with problems were more likely to reply than those without, which, of course, leads to a possible overestimation of the scope of the problem.

Two-thirds of the respondents were women; 85% had been hospitalized at onset of the original polio attack; 95% had experienced paralysis of at least one extremity. Sixty percent were now aged 40–59, median age of 49; 57% had lived with their polio 30–39 years, with a range of 20–74 years. The data revealed that over the decades of the 20th century, the age of onset increased as did the severity of the polio infection in this group. Median age of those who initially required a ventilator was 17, whereas median age of those who did not need ventilator assistance was 9.

Regardless of the severity of the initial polio episode, most respondents achieved some neurological and functional recovery, which reached its maximum 6 years after onset. This recovery lasted a median of 26 years, at which point many respondents noted a decline in health and overall function.

Incidence of wheelchair use illustrates this evolutionary process from onset, through the period of maximum recovery, to the present.

Wheelchair	Onset	Max. recovery	Now
Yes	65%	40%	59%
No	35%	60%	41%

Apparently some who never needed a wheelchair initially must now use one in addition to the many who were able to give up the chair for an extended period of time. New health problems reported include:

Fatigue	87%
Weakness in previously affected muscles	81%
Muscle pain	75%
Joint pain	75%
Weakness in previously unaffected muscles	71%
Breathing difficulties	42%

These health problems have been accompanied by new difficulties in walking, climbing stairs, bathing, and transfers.

The fatigue was described as a pervasive exhaustion associated with a reduced level of energy and endurance. As with those with spinal injury, pacing of daily activities and often a reduction in the absolute number of activities was necessary. Thus, conservation of energy has become a prime concern.

The muscle pain is deep and aching, similar to that of the acute polio episode. Rest and reduced activity usually help, as do heat and aspirin. Joint pain was usually associated with activity, and, thus, rest, change of routine, and nonsteroidal antiinflammatory medication helped. Muscle weakness responded best to a reduced activity level. But, as must be obvious, this constellation of problems can seriously alter an active lifestyle with consequent emotional stress. It was the fatigue particularly that finally forced Bill (one of our biographees) to retire and he has noticed increasing muscle weakness even since this rather dramatic curtailment of activities.

Halstead et al. analyzed their data to determine if there was a certain set of variables that could be used to predict who would be most vulnerable to post-polio decline. Severity of the initial polio episode (required hospitalization, required ventilator assistance, and paralysis or paresis of all four limbs) and over age 10 at onset were associated with a higher incidence of post-polio problems by 40 years' duration of disability. Gender was not a factor in their present sample.

Age at onset of the post-polio problems revealed that the largest percentage of respondents experienced problems in the 41–59 year age range, with 85% of the group reporting fatigue and 80% reporting weakness in previously affected muscles.

Other health problems were noted particularly in the group with the most severe initial polio episode (those who were hospitalized) in contrast to those not requiring hospitalization. In the former group, 33% reported hypertension; respiratory disease, 30%; arthritis, 26%; and heart disease, 24%. The incidence of these problems in those not hospitalized with polio was minimal. It will be important to cross-validate these results on a larger and more representative sample and to compare the incidence with the base rates for these disorders in the nondisabled population.

It is important to note that exercise was recommended as a therapy for muscle weakness, but, in many cases, it produced rather disastrous results: it made the problem worse. Thus, persons with the residuals of polio are cautioned to use good judgment in this matter and to seek physicians who know something about this new problem. Generally, a rule of thumb might be to participate in daily activity within reason as a way of maintaining strength and to avoid excessive exercise programs until we learn more about the cause of this weakness (Maynard, 1985).

Various investigators have searched for an explanation for the muscle weakness and fatigue in polio survivors. Tomlinson (1985) reported that nondisabled older persons maintain a normal number of motor neurons in their spinal cords up to age 60, and the numbers decrease by 29% over the *next four decades*, i.e., until the person is 100 years old. Even this does not significantly interfere with activities of daily living. Thus, he concluded that the extent of the problem experienced by polio survivors cannot be explained by the loss of neurons through normal aging provided that the motor neurons in question are indeed normal.

Wiechers (1985) analyzed motor unit function after poliomyelitis and hypothesizes that return of strength after polio onset results from three events: (1) strengthening of normal, unimpaired muscles; (2) the recovery of initially impaired motor neurons; and (3) the reinnervation of muscle fibers left orphaned by the death of their original motor neuron. It is the last case that may be of interest in post-polio decline. Some motor neurons were killed by the initial polio virus, leaving the motor fibers without innervation. However, other motor neurons may have sent out terminal axon sprouts to the orphaned muscle fibers and a new neuromuscular junction may been created. Therefore, a single motor neuron, originally intended to drive 100–500 muscle fibers, might eventually drive 1,000–2,000 fibers. After 20–30 years of this activity, the motor neuron may either lose the ability to drive this many fibers, and/or individual neuromuscular junctions gradually disintegrate so that the number of muscle fibers driven by this motor neuron declines. This is one hypothesis to explain the fatigue and weakness experienced by some individuals with polio.

The term, progressive post-polio muscular atrophy (PPMA), has been used to describe the new muscle weakness that is appearing in the post-polio group. The key word is "new." Is the atrophy occurring now in previously unimpaired motor neurons and fibers or is it the result of previously orphaned motor fibers disintegrating as Wiechers hypothesized? Dalakas et al. (1985) hypothesized that this may be an immunological disturbance or reactivation of the old polio virus. Herbison et al. (1985) have demonstrated experimentally that muscle weakness can be induced by too much exercise over a period of time.

More recently, Dalakas et al. (1986) report on a follow-up study of 27 persons (15 males and 12 females) who had been referred to the National Institute of Neurological and Communicative Disorders and Stroke for PPMA and then were re-evaluated later. Individuals were included if: they had partial recovery of motor function after polio and functional stability of recovery for at least 15 years; they had residual muscle atrophy, weakness, and areflexia in at least one limb but normal sensation; they had new muscle weakness and neuromuscular symptoms that were unrelated to any other neurological or medical disorder. Only persons less than 60 years old at initial visit were included in order to eliminate "normal" aging as a factor in the altered function. Average age at initial visit was 42.7 years; the range was 24–59. Re-evaluations were conducted an average of 8.2 years later (range, 4.5–20). Average age of these participants was now 50.5 years (range, 36–69); average age of onset of new symptoms was 39.6 (range, 25–56); average number of years after acute polio when new symptoms began was 28.8 years (range, 15–54).

Evaluations included neurological exams, blood chemistry and spinal fluid analyses, electromyography, nerve-conduction studies, and open-muscle biopsy of currently affected muscles. Quantitative assessment of muscle function was accomplished using the Medical Research Council rating scale.

All persons had evidence of PPMA with new muscle weakness and atrophy involving muscles previously affected and fully or partly recovered or muscles that were clinically unaffected by the original disease. The new weakness was asymmetrical and often associated with increasing muscle atrophy. Some experienced muscle pain. All patients were weaker at follow-up and had a lower level of function, but the changes occurred very slowly and varied both across and within individuals. Some had episodes of decline followed by relative stability and some had a slow, steady decline in strength. Those who had been followed the longest had more decline than those followed a shorter time; however, the rate of decline each year was the same in both groups. Generally, the new weakness was so mild that it was not noticeable on a yearly basis, but over a period of years the effect became obvious.

None of the 27 individuals had amyotrophic lateral sclerosis (ALS). Age of onset of new symptoms, gender, and degree and type of physical activities before new weakness appeared were not factors in the progression of the problem.

Dalakas et al. endorse Wiechers' hypothesis that deterioration of individual nerve terminals in PPMA might be the result of recovery from the original polio attack. That is, surviving motor neurons sprout to reinnervate more muscle fibers than normal. This produces large motor units that stress the cell body. Over time, these overfunctioning motor neurons with their excessive sprouting may not be able to handle the demands of their sprouts and a slow deterioration of the individual terminals may result. Dalakas et al. suggest that some individual fibers may be able to be reinnervated a second time, but over time enough nerve terminals are destroyed and weakness appears. This accounts for the slow, stepwise, unpredictable progression. This cannot be explained by normal aging because of the age of these study subjects.

The authors are unable to clarify the roles of virological or immunological mechanisms in PPMA. *They did not find evidence of antibodies to the polio virus, which suggests that there is not a reactivation of the original polio infection as some have feared.* However, they did find some antibodies, suggesting the possibility of some kind of an immunological process in these persons with PPMA that were not found in individuals not experiencing PPMA after the initial attack of polio. Thus, much research is needed to clarify the entire issue of PPMA.

It is very important to note that Dalakas' study (1986), while representing good research technique, deals with a limited sample of persons: those already identified as having PPMA. The pattern and extent of new muscle weakness was highly individualized, and, therefore, it is impossible to generalize these results, at this time, to other individuals with the residuals of polio. Furthermore, it must be emphasized that we do not know what percentage of the post-polio population exhibits PPMA, and, consequently, the scope of the difficulty has not been ascertained.

Furthermore, it is important to note that the etiology of the muscle weakness experienced by some of our post-polio group continues to be controversial at this point, and there is a tremendous amount of research that needs to be done.

Osteoporosis may or may not be or become a problem in the polio group because a large percentage of individuals has been ambulatory. However, it would be important to monitor this with increasing age in this group and in those whose mobility is declining.

The polio group were themselves pioneers along with the spinal injury group. There were few people with disabilities visible in society before the polio epidemics of the 1940s and early 1950s, and, therefore, they had few role models of how to be disabled. As a result, they blended into "nondisabled" society and have very successfully disappeared into the activities of everyday life. They have placed great demands on themselves in many cases for extraordinary performance, demands to accomplish as much as "nondisabled" peers in careers, families, and communities. But the extra energy and expense required to accomplish this feat has also taken its toll. The average person with polio residuals has not used a wheelchair, has had muscle function of some amount in the lower extremities, and as a result, has had the opportunity to overuse the functional muscles to an even greater extent than people paralyzed with spinal injury who are required to use a wheelchair. Thus, Selye's theory of physiological stress (discussed below), Wiechers' hypothesis of overextended motor neurons, and Herbison's observations of muscle destruction from too much exercise of normal muscles may in combination provide a viable explanation of the current difficulties being experienced by this group.

Some people have raised the question as to why we should spend time and money to research aging issues in our post-polio group. One could view it as a self-limiting problem that will disappear when these polio survivors pass away. However, our post-polio people are aging human systems with some problems common to all aging groups and some problems possibly relevant to other neuromuscular diseases. Consequently, whether the muscle weakness, pain, and fatigue are truly unique to polio has not been established. Does this pattern exist in other neuromuscular diseases? Can we truly believe that we will never have another epidemic of polio, and, therefore, do not need to research the consequences of this disease?

MULTIPLE SCLEROSIS

Multiple sclerosis is a neurological disorder in which the myelin sheath of the nerve fiber deteriorates and the transmission of the electrical impulse along the nerve fiber is interrupted at this point. The etiology of this disorder is unknown and there is no known cure at this time. The myelin may or may not regenerate, and, if not, a sclera or scar remains that impedes the nerve impulse at that point, resulting in neurological impairment. Any one or combination of nerves can be affected, and, therefore, the pattern of symptoms varies across individuals with this disorder. Since the myelin sheath disintegrates and recovers in a truly unpredictable pattern, the disorder is characterized by exacerbations and remissions of neurological symptoms over time. Thus, not only is there variability as to which nerves may be affected, but the seriousness of the symptoms and timing and pattern of recovery or deterioration are dissimilar from one person to another. Unfortunately, one of the only similarities among individuals with multiple sclerosis is a sense of anxiety about the future because of the unpredictablity of the evolution of the disorder.

Obviously, there is a variety of ways in which people cope with this unpredictability, and most people learn to take each day at a time and try not to dwell on potential problems in the future. It is often difficult to plan ahead with any certainty, however, and this feature of the disorder is certainly a source of major stress.

Since there is such tremendous variability of physical and sensory impairments associated with multiple sclerosis, there does not seem to be any typical pattern of aging. These individuals may be vulnerable to many of the difficulties experienced by those with other long-term physical disabilities, such as reduced energy, the potential for musculoskeletal problems, and the "diseases of civilization." Some clinicians have speculated that the disease may "burn out" with age, i.e., it stabilizes at a certain level of dysfunction and the pattern of exacerbations and remissions disappears. If this proves to be the case, it will be ironic that people with multiple sclerosis will be able to experience for the first time some degree of certainty in their lives at the point that others with seemingly more "static" disabilities are becoming overwhelmed by the uncertainty of the course of their physical function. However, even if the multiple sclerosis itself stabilizes, there may still be aging problems associated with long-term disability, plus normal aging as a continuing fact of life. Consequently, there is a great deal of research that needs to be done before we will understand the aging process in those with multiple sclerosis and other progressive neurological disorders.

DISABILITIES OF CONGENITAL OR CHILDHOOD ONSET

Individuals with cerebral palsy, spina bifida, and other disabilities acquired at birth or in childhood have also experienced "aging" problems that are particularly noticeable in the musculoskeletal system. Pain, soreness, weakness of muscles, and energy decline have been reported along with the tendency to be increasingly susceptible to injury as noted above among those with spinal injury and residuals of polio. Scoliosis and spinal deformities are especially noticeable in those who acquired a disability at an early age. These difficulties are detectable when the individuals are in their 20s and 30s, which can become a major psychosocial crisis. After striving throughout childhood and teenage years to achieve success in school, work, friendships, and family, the opportunity to enjoy the rewards may seem prematurely challenged by altered or declining function. After having worked toward independent living and to be free of parents, one's whole world could be threatened by the need for more assistance or the need to reduce level of activity. It is not easy to experience this in one's late 40s or 50s, but in one's early adult years the situation may seem terribly unjust and grim at times. Thus, the issue of aging with a disability is not necessarily associated with one's chronological age but rather seems to be correlated with time since onset of the disability. Twenty to thirty years in an active person will produce wear and tear on the musculoskeletal system in general and other body systems depending on the lifestyle of the person, one's genetic heritage, and the nature of the disability.

HEALTH PROBLEMS COMMON TO MANY DISABILITIES

Musculoskeletal Problems

Most of the persons with a major physical disability of at least 30 years' duration note some tenderness and soreness in the joints, muscles, and tendons, which have been carrying the extra burden of impaired physical function in other parts of the body. Furthermore, osteoporosis has complicated the lives of certain of my informants as bones become increasingly brittle with age.

The wrist is particularly vulnerable to injury, arthritis, or carpal tunnel syndrome (CTS) as a result of use of crutches in those who ambulate or transfers and wheelchair propulsion in those who do not walk. Aljure et al. (1985) studied the incidence of CTS in 47 persons with paraplegia of T2 or lower. Electromyography (EMG) was performed to assess conduction in the median and ulnar nerves. Duration of injury ranged from 3 months to 42 years and was highly correlated with incidence of CTS (Table 4-1). Twenty-four persons did not report signs or symptoms of CTS and/or ulnar nerve disease; of those, 16 had normal test results; eight had abnormal EMGs.

It appears that extended use of certain body parts to compensate for lost motor ability can lead to problems over time. This is the only study available that examines this issue explicitly; thus, we can only speculate that other joints

Table 4-1. *Incidence of CTS in 47 Persons with Paraplegia*

Duration of disability	No. persons (hands)	Clinical CTS (hands)	Percent CTS
1 year	2 (4)	0 (0)	0
1–5	10 (20)	3 (6)	30
6–10	5 (10)	3 (3)	30
11–20	11 (22)	7 (12)	54
21–30	7 (13)	5 (7)	54
31+	12 (22)	12 (20)	90
Total	47 (91)	30 (48)	63

would experience similar dysfunctions over time. Soreness in shoulders and neck has often been reported by my sample, in addition to wrist difficulties. As a result, many are altering their equipment and mobility techniques to reduce discomfort and to prevent further problems. Some have adopted the new lightweight wheelchairs, but many have opted for electric wheelchairs, which require the additional expense of van with hydraulic lift if this chair is to be the primary mode of mobility. Many who were ambulatory have now begun to use a wheelchair, and sliding boards for transfers are being adopted by some. A majority of the musculoskeletal problems are reported by those with paraplegia or quadriplegia who transfer independently. Higher-level quadriplegics report little or no difficulty with these problems, apparently because these body parts were not able to perform such physically abusive tasks. This observation, however, must be assessed by future research.

Declining energy and strength seems also to be associated with an increase in injuries to tendons and muscles from transferring. These injuries can be frustrating and exceedingly disruptive to function for certain periods of time. Thus, many persons with long-term disability re-examine their techniques and often alter their mobility strategies to prevent future problems. One person recommended using a variety of transfer techniques so as to distribute the stress across different muscles and tendons. Most have become very resourceful at assessing their energy expenditure in a typical day and taking steps to prioritize how they will expend their energy. This may involve home modifications (such as a roll-in shower), purchase of other equipment (electric wheelchair, van and lift, electric bed), and, almost universally, a reduction in the number of events scheduled during a day or week. *Energy conservation and further disability prevention have become a major factor in each of my informants' lives.*

The decision to accept more adaptive equipment is not easily reached. Those who have been ambulatory find it very difficult to accept a wheelchair or motorized device part-time or full-time. Others resist the electric wheelchair and van until they are in such discomfort that their daily lives become depressingly constricted. But even after making the change, the thought may persist that one has failed, that one has "given in" to the disability. For years, these individuals were confronted by people who said, "You can't do that," so that it is almost a reflex reaction to respond, "Oh, yes I can!" Consequently, we must remember that all of those with disabilities of 30 or more years represent our pioneers, people who refused to give in to the image of disability as invalidism in the early days. Thus, in some respects these individuals have "out-normaled" the "normals." Some people might use the term overachievers, but that concept has never made any sense to me; it implies that one has achieved more than one was supposed to achieve! These people are merely great achievers. Consequently, it is exceedingly important that professionals tread lightly when proposing that someone with long-term disability change the way that he or she does things, especially if it means using additional equipment. A period of consultation, advice, reflection, and gentle persuasion may be necessary along with the realization that some will continue to aggravate a condition until they have absolutely no choice but to change. Rather than perceiving this as obstinacy and stupidity, it can just as easily be viewed as resiliency, strength, and self-determination, all very admirable traits. At this point, it is interesting to recall that Clifford continued to walk until his hip joints literally would not support him anymore, and after 12 years he still considers the wheelchair to represent giving in to the disability. In fact, it is almost as if it represents the onset of disability to him.

The spine itself may become a focal point for difficulty because of scoliosis or certain arthritic and osteoporotic changes. Those who acquired the disability during their growing years of childhood are particularly vulnerable, as well as those with incomplete spinal injury and the residuals of polio. Pain frequently becomes the problem; it limits function and requires adaptation in mobility techniques and equipment. One of my informants believes that the entire body gradually goes out of alignment as bones and joints slightly rearrange their position in regard to each other. Whether or not this is widespread in incidence or has a significant impact on function remains to be seen.

Increasing bone fractures have been noted in some, and particularly in women. Post-menopausal women are more vulnerable to osteoporosis than men of equal age and the presence of a physical disability may aggravate the problem because of restricted mobility. Yet, calcium loss is a frequent concomitant of spinal injury; thus, the incidence of osteoporosis in physically disabled men and women in contrast to their "nondisabled" counterparts would be an important issue to assess. Does this increase with age at the same rate in both sexes and with duration of disability? What is the effect of participation in athletics on osteoporosis in people with disabilities? Is the effect, if present, similar in men and women? What is the effect of calcium supplements? Is this effective in both men and women? In what doses? What impact do calcium supplements have on bladder and kidney function? Does exercise to prevent osteoporosis and to increase cardiovascular conditioning accelerate the rate of energy loss and joint dysfunction in long-term disability?

Certainly, a survey of the normal SCI and post-polio populations (not hospitalized ones) is in order to assess the incidence of these various difficulties according to current age, duration of disability, gender, current and previous activity level, level of SCI, previous history of athletic participation, and excess body weight. An interesting question is whether active and consistent participation in sports accelerates musculoskeletal difficulties or retards them because of overall physical condition and health. What steps, if any, can be taken in the earlier years of disability to prevent or reduce musculoskeletal problems? What is the effect of excess body weight on the development of these disorders?

Any research should use "nondisabled" control groups matched on the above variables, since arthritis is the most frequently reported disability in aging Americans (*Aging America*, 1984). For every 1,000 persons, 246 report arthritic problems in the 45–64 age group, and 465 report such problems at 65 years and over. Osteoporosis studies must pay particular attention to the issue of age and gender and use "nondisabled" control groups in order to provide any useful information. Thus, there are numerous studies that need to be done to elucidate the above issues.

Nutrition and Exercise

There is increasing evidence that the lifestyle, particularly the eating and exercise habits, of the American public is a factor in our diseases of civilization. As a result, persons with disabilities are as vulnerable, if not more vulnerable, to these problems. Reduced mobility and energy with age, plus the stress of the disability, may compound the deleterious impact of a high-fat, high-protein, high-sugar diet. Perhaps an alteration of the nutritional habits of those with long-term disability might modulate the problems of aging. For example, high complex carbohydrate, low-fat diets have produced great energy, health, and physical performance in athletes. Could such a diet modulate the long-term impact of aging with a disability and additionally reduce the incidence of cardiovascular disorders? One could speculate that the additional physical burdens imposed by paralysis every day are similar to an athletic event, but those with disabilities have not viewed it as such and therefore have not "trained" for the great sport of surviving with the disability, other than making it through the initial rehabilitation program. It is quite apparent that I do not consider the body to be a machine, yet what we ingest does serve as a fuel; it does provide the energy and nutrients that individual cells need to perform their tasks. The body is very resilient; neverthelsss, we may be able to optimize this metabolic process by giving the body what it needs in order to perform at peak efficiency. In paraplegia, for example, the upper half of the body is asked to do the work normally performed by the lower half. Discus, shotput, and javelin throwers take great pains to get in shape and eat correctly. Yet, most with paraplegia continue to eat and exercise as if they had the entire body working for them. Those without disabilities who have been athletic all of their lives and who have continued to eat and exercise properly seem to age less rapidly and are healthier than their nonathletic counterparts. Even those nonathletes who expend 2,000 calories a week in exercise have been shown to have lower death rates than more sedentary individuals (Paffembarger et al., 1986). Thus, would there be a less noticeable decline in energy and fewer musculoskeletal and cardiovascular problems in those who stayed in "training" during their life with the disability? Would they be less vulnerable to pressure sores because of general good health and the type of food being consumed? Would the disability take less of a toll over the years from mental stress because the exercise and type of food ingested enhanced a sense of well-being? Would a daily dose of endorphins have a positive impact on daily function of those with disabilities as it does for runners and other regularly active people?

If one considers the physical demands of disability to be somewhat like an athletic event (only this one lasts a lifetime), physical conditioning, whether or not one is interested in sports, may be an added advantage in coping with the physical disability. Perhaps the decline in energy and strength has been accelerated by performing in repeated athletic events (activities of daily living and mobility) without being in proper physical condition. One need not pump iron, but regular muscle and cardiovascular conditioning may offset some of this decline.

While not considered medical problems, the issues of nutrition and exercise in long-term disability are fertile avenues of research for those interested in the health care of those with physical disability.

Stress and the Endocrine System

The endocrine system plays a powerful role in regulating the homeostasis, the equilibrium, of the body. Claus-Walker and Halstead (1981, 1982a–d) have accomplished the herculean task of reviewing all of the literature on endocrine function in SCI in the last 25 years (as of 1981) and they have concisely summarized the results and suggested directions for future research. Since the majority of this information applies to alteration in endocrine function in the early stages of SCI, it will not be reviewed here, but professionals are strongly encouraged to familiarize themselves with this information because there are literally hundreds of research projects relevant to long-term SCIs implicit in these articles. The basic questions are: Do these alterations in endocrine function persist over time? Do they change in format? How do these alterations, if they persist, influence long-term function?

As we consider the endocrine system in long-term disability, Hans Selye, M.D. (1956, 1976) has devoted a lifetime to the study of stress, and much of this research may contain clues to the varied pattern of decline experienced by people with long-term disability. Selye states:

> In its medical sense, *stress is essentially the rate of wear and tear in the body.* Anyone who feels that whatever he is doing—or whatever is being done to him—is strenuous and wearing, knows vaguely what we mean by *stress.* But stress does not necessarily

imply a morbid change: normal life, especially intense pleasure and the ecstasy of fulfillment, also cause some wear and tear on the machinery of the body. Indeed, stress can even have a curative value, as in shock therapy, bloodletting, and sports. In any event, wear and tear is only the result of all this: hence, we now define stress as *the nonspecific response of the body to any demand.*

The nervous and endocrine systems play particularly important roles in maintaining resistance during stress, he hypothesizes, because stress causes certain structural and chemical changes in the body, some signs of damage, some signs of adaptation to stress. Thus, he describes the general adaptation syndrome (GAS), which has three stages: (1) alarm reaction, (2) stage of resistance, and (3) stage of exhaustion. Selye further discusses the concept of adaptation energy to describe that which is consumed during continuous adaptive work but which is other than caloric energy received from food.

It is as though, at birth, each individual inherited a certain amount of adaptation energy, the magnitude of which is determined by one's genetic background, one's parents. He can draw upon this capital thriftily for a long but monotonously uneventful existence, or he can spend it lavishly in the course of a stressful, intense, but perhaps more colorful and exciting life. In any case, there is just so much of it, and he must budget accordingly (p. 82).

Consequently, Selye's stress theory may have great relevance to the process of aging in those with physical disabilities. His GAS is typically applied to an individual stress event, but over a lifetime of living with disability, there may be an early alarm reaction, followed by a lengthy period of resistance or adaptation, but succeeded by exhaustion as adaptation energy is less available.

Although this dedicated researcher has devoted a lifetime to studying the specifics of the stress concept and GAS, we give only a superficial overview of the issue and recommend that anyone interested in aging and disability read Selye's work for a fuller discussion of the topic.

In tissues more directly affected by any individual stress event, there develops a local adaptation syndrome (LAS), for example, inflammation resulting from microbes entering the body. LAS and GAS are closely coordinated, and chemical alarm signals are sent out directly from stressed tissues, from the LAS area to the coordination centers in the nervous system and then to the endocrine glands, especially the pituitary and adrenals. These produce adaptive hormones to combat wear and tear in the body, thus triggering GAS. The adaptive hormones consist of two groups: anti-inflammatory or glucocorticoid hormones (adrenocorticotropic hormone, cortisone, cortisol), which inhibit excessive defensive reactions, and the pro-inflammatory and/or mineralocorticoid hormones (somatotropic hormone, aldosterone, and desoxycorticosterone), which stimulate them.

Collectively, these hormones are called syntoxic because they facilitate coexistence with a pathogen, either by diminishing sensitivity to it or by encapsulating it within a barricade of inflammatory tissue. These must be distinguished from the catatoxic hormones, which promote destruction of potential pathogens through induction of poison-metabolizing enzymes in the liver. The effects of all these substances can be modified or conditioned by other hormones (adrenalines or thyroid hormones), nervous reactions, diets, heredity, and tissue memories of previous exposure to stress.

Consequently, the response to stress consists of the (1) direct effect of the stressor on the body, (2) internal responses that stimulate tissue defenses or help to destroy damaging substances, and (3) internal responses that cause tissue surrender by inhibiting unnecessary or excessive defense. Resistance and adaptation depend on a proper *balance* of these three factors.

Selye discusses the impact of long-term stress, or long-term GAS, on a variety of conditions that he labels "diseases of adaptation," some resulting from an excessive bodily defensive reaction and others from an overabundance of submissive bodily reactions. Therefore, he believes that excessive or insufficient corticoid production influences hypertension, disease of the heart and blood vessels, kidney problems, arthritis, inflammatory diseases of the skin and eyes, infections, allergic and hypersensitivity diseases, nervous and digestive problems, cancer, and diseases of resistance in general. Should we add to this list the decline that persons with long-term disability may experience after 30 years with a disability?

It is of interest to note that Claus-Walker and Halstead (1982c) report altered endocrinological reactions to stress in early SCI and indicate that a lack of secretion of anti-inflammatory steroids, which has been noted in several studies, may play a role in generating pressure sores. Many of my informants describe patterns of problems that might be unified under the concept of reduction of total adaptive energy available or the beginnings of exhaustion. Thus, the GAS concept may be applicable to the totality of life after onset of major physical disability. Perhaps the later years are characterized by a slowly evolving stage of exhaustion that makes one vulnerable to a variety of seemingly unrelated difficulties. This might explain the onset of sudden mysterious internal abscesses and infections that have been noted in some cases; the increased susceptibility to pressure sores in some individuals; a slight increase in bladder cancer over that found in a nondisabled population; the slight increase of cardiovascular disorders in the middle age groups in contrast to the general public; the sudden increase in allergies that Dave reported; and the generalized decline in mental and physical energy.

The issue of Selye's stress theory and the role of endocrine function is equally applicable in these instances of decline of function in polio as well as SCI. The increased incidence of cardiovascular and arthritic problems in those with more severe early episodes of polio certainly correlates with Selye's theory. Those with more severe earlier episodes of polio have survived with greater residual damage, which has imposed greater strain on the body than those with less severe early episodes. The physiological results of stress as wear and tear may indeed be a common denominator in all categories of physical disability, but some of the specific manifestations of this wear and tear will depend on the disability, i.e., every body has its vulnerabilities of one or more organ systems. In polio survivors, the weak point may be the previously orphaned muscle fibers that have been innervated by other motor neurons (resulting in an overworked motor neuron). Furthermore, joints then become increasingly vulnerable to injury and damage as the number of motor fibers gradually declines, with resulting muscle weakness. Previously compromised respiratory function may become more compromised with the passage of time. And most important, the lifetime physiological reserves of energy may be utilized at a faster rate in the process of living with polio than without a disability.

Miscellaneous Health Problems

Throughout this chapter, we have described a number of biological–organic (O) problems in some depth. However, there are several others that deserve to be mentioned and considered for future research and current clinical management.

Dependent edema is a major problem for some individuals and not for others. Why? The lower extremities have been the site of excessive and long-term swelling in a number of my informants so that some have had great problems in finding shoes that fit, do not aggrevate the problem by causing pressure sores, and are cosmetically acceptable if not totally pleasing. This latter may be a particular issue for women because shoes designed for them have never emphasized function or comfort and those that do are sometimes downright ugly. A further concern is whether dependent edema, over time, aggravates or complicates any circulatory problems that the individual may have. In addition, do edematous extremities become the site of blood clot formation and thus increase the probability of pulmonary embolism, cerebrovascular accident, or thrombophlebitis? Do wrappings or elastic hose reduce the problem?

Some individuals have reported a prolapsed rectum or rectal fistula, but this may be more common in those with impaired bowel function. It is possible that 30 or more years of various bowel management programs may produce mechanical damage in the rectal area, which may require surgical repair or even a colostomy. Is the incidence of rectal cancer in those with disabilities any different from that found in the general public of similar age?

The sudden or gradual onset of unusual infections or abscesses has been reported by some. The site of these problems varies, but the circumstances seem similar: an abscess forms in an unexpected location and often requires surgical repair and powerful antibiotics. Is this related to a gradual decline in the endocrine system, in the immune system, so that one is more vulnerable to bacteria that have always been present but not problematical previously?

Hypertension is a significant problem in the general public; however, a number of my informants seem to be experiencing this disorder also. Does the long-term stress of the disability increase the probability that an individual will develop this complication? Does the incidence exceed that in the "nondisabled" population of comparable age?

Many in the post-polio group are certainly noticing an alteration of their respiratory function with age, especially if bulbar symptoms were part of the initial polio attack. Many are finding that their physicians quickly think in terms of a tracheostomy and/or respirator. However, there are a variety of intermediate steps to improve oxygenation that can be utilized prior to such a drastic step. Improper oxygenation at night often becomes a problem that influences overall efficiency and function during the day, and, thus, this compounds the effects of declining energy. How much of the sense of declining energy and fatigue is associated with improper oxygenation either during the day or night?

In our spinal injury group, those with quadriplegia or high-level paraplegia have few or no chest muscles and have relied on diaphragmatic breathing for most of their life with the disability. Certainly, because of this, they have always been vulnerable to respiratory infections, but does proper oxygenation become a problem over the years also?

Osteoporosis has been mentioned earlier but should be considered within this context. A number of my informants have had recent experience of a bone breaking when little force was applied. In the "nondisabled" population, women are more vulnerable to osteoporosis than men, but is this the case for those with disabilities also? Do calcium supplements help? What effect do these supplements have on bladder and kidney stone formation?

Individuals with long-term disability may over the years acquire quite a pharmacopoeia that they must ingest daily. Medications for spasticity, hypertension, and genitourinary conditions are frequently prescribed, and we do not know the effects of long-term usage of these in combination as the person ages. We have evidence that the "efficiency" of body function declines with age. Does this alter the effect and potency of some drugs? What happens when new medications are added to the list? Not only do we not have sufficient research on this issue, we probably do not have sufficient attention being given to the possibility of drug interaction side-effects in the clinical management of individuals with long-term disability.

PREVENTION

And now we come to the issue of prevention, certain aspects of which are discussed in the section on nutrition and exercise, and thus those parameters will not be mentioned here. But a burning question is: Does voluntary curtailment in the intensity and scope of activities at an earlier age translate into fewer musculoskeletal difficulties in the later years? One friend remained an avid outdoorsman after onset of his spinal injury and derived immense pleasure from kayaking and other sports activities. At one point, when he was experiencing the first twinges of discomfort in his neck and shoulders, his physician commented, "If you have one million muscle contractions remaining, would you rather use them for kayaking or for transferring?" At the time, my friend thought that this was a terrible thing to say to a person, but now he realizes that there was some wisdom in that question. However, outdoor activities were so essential to his sense of well-being that he could not seriously consider any curtailment in this area. Even though he now has had to limit his sports activities to a minimum in order to conserve his energy, he does not regret his passionate involvement with the outdoors, but he certainly mourns their loss. If he had done half as much, would he have had twice as long to participate in these activities? How do we convince a passionately committed and dynamic person to do less than he or she is capable of or wants to do? Should we try?

Such issues confront many of our polio survivors who have ambulated with braces and crutches for many years. Before they experience significant difficulties, should they begin using a wheelchair at least part of the time? Everyone needs their arms and hands for daily activities, but those whose arms and fingers are essential to their vocation, such as a draftsman or artist, might need to consider the tradeoff of ambulation versus arm function. Is this wise anticipatory planning or unnecessary neurotic worrying? Unfortunately, because of the lack of incidence studies, we do not know.

It is certainly in the area of prevention that we need some high-quality prospective clinical research in our younger population of persons with disabilities. Longitudinal studies on the role of exercise, cardiopulmonary conditioning, nutrition, active participation in sports, and pacing of the intensity and variety of physical activities need to be conducted.

RATE AND FORMAT OF THE AGING PROCESS

As we have reviewed the issue of aging with a disability, it has become clear that there is little definitive knowledge available at this time, but we have identified a multitude of questions that should be the focus of future research. From the literature reviewed and the information volunteered by the persons interviewed for this book, it seems likely that the musculoskeletal system is particularly vulnerable to further disability after 20–40 years of living with a physical disability. When a delimited number of muscles, tendons, and joints are asked to perform the work of a larger number, it seems reasonable that the extra work may lead to wear and tear sooner than if they had not been placed under extra stress. The degree of musculoskeletal dysfunction seems to be associated with the amount of extra labor, the duration of this extra labor, one's general physical condition and health, and one's genetic heritage. As a result, those who have been very physically active seem to be experiencing difficulties with this body system. Whether this applies equally to those who have been consistently involved in sports activities will have to be determined. Furthermore, the issue of physical conditioning for this extra labor may be a powerful factor in ameliorating the impact of long-term stress on this body system.

Also, we have noted, both within the spinal injury and post-polio group, an incidence of cardiovascular problems when people are in their 40s that may be greater than that experienced by a "nondisabled" group of similar age. Whether or not one experiences such problems will be correlated with family history and lifestyle factors, but the physical, emotional, and financial stress of a physical disability may be reflected in this body system in those predisposed to cardiovascular disorders. The endocrine system may be generally vulnerable, regardless of the disability, if Selye's stress theory of alarm, resistance, and exhaustion describes the lifetime physiological process of living with a physical disability.

Thus, it may be true that living with a major physical disability, regardless of the type of disability, leads to a decline in certain bodily systems in certain individuals sooner than if they had not been disabled. However, it seems probable that there will be tremendous variability across individuals even within the same disability group based on differences in lifestyle, genetics, health habits, and physical activity level. It is important to note that some individuals, whether disabled or "nondisabled," age very gracefully and others seem to "age" early. Consequently, there will be tremendous heterogeneity within the population of persons with physical disability.

Based on the limited information available, we do not have evidence at this time that the rate of aging is different for various disabilities. Rather, at this point, the amount of time after onset seems to be the major variable, and, even within this, there is tremendous variability across people (20–40 years of disability).

The format of the aging process seems to have some similarities that cut across all disabilities and some unique features that may be associated with specific disabilities. As we have discussed, the generalized wear and tear of living with a disability seems to be reflected in the musculoskeletal, cardiovascular, and endocrine systems. However, those with spinal injury or polio may be susceptible to certain additional dysfunctions. The genitourinary system is a focal point for potential problems in spinal injury, and muscle weakness and atrophy in previously functional muscles seems to be unique to polio. The muscle pain and degree of fatigue that individuals with polio residuals report seem to be greater than that experienced by those with spinal injury. However, whether this is related to the event of the poliomyelitis itself or related to the greater amount of physical acitivity in which many with polio residuals have engaged remains to be determined through further research. Additionally, some of those with polio residuals who required ventilator support during the acute phase are now noticing a decline in vital capacity. Spinal-injured persons with high-level quadriplegia have always been vulnerable to respiratory infections, but whether or not respiratory function declines with age is not known. Here again, there will be a great degree of variability across individuals based on lifestyle, genetic heritage, and environmental resources.

As decribed in Chapter 3, aging with a disability is a continuation of the process of adjusting to a disability, a psychosocial, biological–organic, environmental (P,O,E) balance. The issue of aging becomes noticeable when there is a change in the biological–organic (O) component of our human system that tips the balance, so to speak, requiring a readjustment in the psychosocial (P) and environmental (E) variables in order to achieve an equilibrium again. It is now to these psychosocial and environmental variables that we turn in an effort to understand the complexity of the process of aging with a disability.

5

The Psychological and Environmental Implications of Aging

BACK TO THE BALANCING ACT

People who have lived with a physical disability for 30 or more years have long ago joined the group that we label as having "adjusted to the disability." Yet, what is adjustment? How many people who are reading this book, whether disabled or "nondisabled," consider themselves to be adjusted? Adjusted to what? Adjustment is not a static condition that has a definable start and endpoint; furthermore, it does not exist in a vacuum. Rather, adjustment is an evolutionary process in all of our lives and we are always in the process of adjusting to our internal and external environments. Thus, adjustment is synonymous with the balancing act we perform every day as we seek equilibrium among our emotional state, our bodily condition, and the environment in which we live, the P,O,E system. *We, humans, are P,O,E systems, and all of our behavior, everything that we do and feel, are reflections of this P,O,E system.*

The early years after disability onset are devoted to using one's pyschosocial (P) resources to shape and accommodate to an environment (E) that permits maximum function given the constraints imposed by the disability on bodily function (O). It may take up to five years or even longer to accommodate to the changes required and to create for oneself a life worth living. Every body has its weak points, and the disability may impose additional weak points, which people with disabilities learn to accommodate. Consequently, those who manage this balancing act for 30 or more years are extremely resourceful, strong, self-reliant, and knowledgable people and may now find themselves facing the second onset of disability in some cases—a decline in physical function that unbalances the P,O,E equilibrium. The decline in physical function influences one's perception of oneself (P) and one's access to satisfying and rewarding activities (E), both of which can have a powerful impact on mood. Furthermore, the changes in biological–organic (O) functioning may require environmental changes, such as the need for more help from family or hired assistance, more adaptive equipment, a different living environment, perhaps. As a result, these changes also impact on mood, which, of course, influences bodily function.

Aging is a part of living that forces one to adjust to the ever-changing internal and external environments. In the previous chapter, we presented a variety of hypotheses as to the nature of the biological–organic (O) changes a person with a major physical disability might experience over time. Now we need to look at the impact of these organic changes on the psychosocial (P) and environmental (E) parameters of one's human system.

PSYCHOSOCIAL (P) IMPACT OF THE AGING PROCESS

Acceptance of Responsibility

Anyone who survives 30 or more years with a major physical disability has long ago accepted responsibility for his or her own life. Bodies with disabilities need extra care in order to keep functioning, and the environment has presented social and physical obstacles on a daily basis that had to be surmounted. Those unwilling or unable to meet the challenge probably died a long time ago, either of active or passive suicide.

Passive suicide occurs by not accepting responsibility and allowing the biological and environmental variables to get so extremely out of balance that one eventually dies of "legitimate" medical conditions. In the early days of acute disability management, medical problems killed a large number of people who wanted to live, either because their bodies had too many weak points or their environment was very unsupportive. However, the lack of medical knowledge was also a convenient opportunity to let nature take its course, so to speak; thus, in the early days, it was easier to die legitimately if one was not committed to living. This hypothesis derives from the increased incidence of active suicide reported in the most recent longevity-mortality study from Toronto (Geisler et al., 1983). Suicide accounted for 10.8% of the deaths in the sample between 1973 and 1980, whereas it was a cause of death in 4.2% of the deaths prior to 1973. As noted in Chapter 3, this study added many recent injuries to the sample between 1973 and 1980, which may explain the changed incidence. Given the advances in current disability management techniques, it may be less easy to die naturally, and, therefore, more definitive steps need to be taken to withdraw from the battle. An alternative hypothesis is that more older persons with major disabilities are actively choosing to end their lives in this manner. This is not an impossibility, but it is certainly inconsistent with a lifetime history of survival. If we had data on cause of death by age group and era of early SCI management, this issue would not be such a mystery.

Consequently, the lifetime experience of accepting responsiblity for one's own life and creating a life worth living gives one a sense of self-reliance and self-confidence; the belief that one can take care of oneself. Furthermore, as our biographies have demonstrated, most of these individuals have adopted the philosophy of self-reliance *because* you cannot count on anyone else. They may count heavily on their wives (not many older disabled women have husbands to count on), but, nevertheless, they rely on their own native ingenuity and energy to get things done. Mastery of the disability means having achieved an equilibrium in their P,O,E system. But as their biological–organic function changes, the equilibrium is disrupted and their sense of self-reliance and self-confidence is threatened, which leads to turmoil until some semblance of equilibrium is achieved again. The sense of self-reliance is threatened by the fear of loss of independence—the necessity of having to count on someone else to get the job done. The declining function and energy threatens the lifetime self-confidence that one can handle anything that comes along. Unfortunately, these fears are not myths or the result of "neuroses," but rather are accurately based in reality and, thus, there is no easy remedy.

Dave, after a lifetime of living alone, is worried about his ability to handle the future by himself, and, thus, has gotten married, which introduces new stresses. Other men in my sample have acquired wives (quite a bit younger than themselves) recently or have contemplated that option seriously. Consequently, the formation of a new family is one option to solve the problem of loss of independence; unfortunately, this option is not as readily available to disabled women because men seem to be less tolerant of physical impairments in women.

Frank was psychologically devastated by the six-month immobilization in the hospital after a lifetime of almost perfect health. Therefore, the very process of treatment within the sickness treatment system can undermine one's sense of confidence and self-reliance (Trieschmann, 1984a). Interactions with the sickness treatment system are usually fraught with frustration and anger. After managing one's own body successfully, people with long-term disability must cope with young people just out of medical residency (or still in it) who peremptorily announce that one's medication *will be* changed (even though the person had determined by continuing self-analysis and evaluation that just that medication works correctly for him or her); one's self-care procedure *must be* changed; or a certain diagnostic or treatment procedure *will be* given. All of these decisions are often made without consultation with the person or recognition that the person is perfectly capable of participating in the decision-making process. The disabled person is frequently disenfranchised from the body that he or she has protected and often removed from the decision-making process by professionals who expect deference to be given to their "superior" knowledge. However, even when the person is consulted about the procedures to be taken, the immobilization itself with its attendant psychological isolation from a normal life is devastating and undermines one's sense of self-confidence. The results of sensory deprivation studies (Zubek, 1969) can easily be generalized to the circumstances of long hospitalizations. The ability to remain in control has been the essence of these people's lives, and the sickness treatment system is totally antithetical to the principle of patient control (Cousins, 1983; Weil, 1983; Trieschmann, 1984*a*).

Thus, it is of paramount importance that all health care professionals approach those with long-term disability with a sense of respect for their accomplishments: they are survivors, not "old crocks." Treat them as you would treat your own mother or father who is experiencing a decline. You respect them for what they have done in their lives and you provide a caring framework in which they keep their self-respect and as much control over their lives as they are *intellectually* able to manage.

The Will to Live

As we have discussed earlier, the will to live is essential to survival with a major physical disability, and most of those without this desire to live succumb to legitimate medical problems or suicide. But most of my informants report a decline in energy that makes them vulnerable to thoughts about the meaning of life. They have fought for life, liberty, and the pursuit of happiness, but many of them are tiring of the battle. Frustrations occur more readily, and they report less energy available to cope with the stress of daily life. Those without financial compensation or high incomes are particularly tired of fighting to barely survive.

Dave, one of the strongest and most self-reliant people that I know, admitted that the thought of suicide has occurred to him lately and it worries him. He is terribly tired of devoting so much energy to mere survival without the hope that things will get better for him and others in similar predicaments. In addition to the loss of hope that things will get better, he is facing the reality that things might get worse, and he fears that he may not have the energy to restore the balance, the equilibrium, in his life as his biological–organic function declines.

Sally and Jack also report being tired of the battle to live. The problem is that these people face an unsupportive environment (at the societal level) that they have overcome only through the expenditure of great personal energy. Now their energy is declining, and they know that their freedom depends on a fight to stay out of a nursing home. Thus, they worry whether they have enough energy left to continue the fight to be free.

Our sickness treatment system is structured so that the easiest solution to aging with a disability is to put these people in a nursing home. Certainly, we do not have enough nursing homes (or the money to support this endeavor) to handle such a population, but neither do we have an alternative in existence at the present time: *a system of support services that automatically keeps people in their own homes until this is no longer feasible.*

Thus, for these people with long-term physical disability (and many without disability) the will to live is strongly associated with the need to be free—to control one's own destiny, to make one's own decisions, and to die with dignity. If we take away their freedom, what impact will this have on the mortality rate? This is an interesting and somewhat macabre question for future research.

Social Skills

Those who have lived a long time with a physical disability have a viable set of social skills that has permitted them to create a reasonable life; to deal with the sickness treatment system and yet survive all of these years; to relate to family, friends, co-workers, and bureaucrats; and to live in an environment designed by and for "nondisabled" people. The resourcefulness, creativity, and knowledge of their own disability have given them a well-deserved sense of self-reliance and self-confidence, which, as they grow older, may be reflected in a tendency to suffer fools less tolerantly.

As all of us get older, we may become cranky, feisty, and less concerned about being nice. We become set in our ways; we become less tolerant of change: change in routine, change in environment, or change in companions. Therefore, as biological function declines, the person may become quite resistant to the new procedures, the new equipment, the new environments (all E variables) required to restore the functional balance. Irascibility, stubbornness, and anger (P variables) may be evident as one attempts to continue the fight to overcome the disability, all of which will make relationships with family, friends, and health care professionals tenuous at times.

As mentioned before, this individual, this expert at living with a disability, will be quite intolerant of health care professionals who exhibit a lack of specialized knowledge *and* a lack of caring for the human being involved. When the professional truly cares, he or she will not hide behind a facade of facts but will be willing to join in partnership with the disabled person to devise an effective strategy to ameliorate the problem. My informants are really quite forgiving of physicians who may not have all of the answers but who sincerely care and demonstrate this by soliciting and respecting the opinion of the disabled person and then proceeding to acquire more information about the problem on their own. On the other hand, people with long-term disability are not happy when the health care professional totally defers to the disabled person's opinion about bodily function as an excuse to avoid getting involved or to cover up a lack of interest in learning more about the problem. Resentment deepens when the professional expects to be paid a fee for nonservice or lack of knowledge. This situation occurs frequently when dealing with physicians who have not been trained in rehabilitation, i.e., a majority of the private practitioners in any community. However, our older disabled group has also run into this problem among specialists who focus on acute physical medicine rather than long-term rehabilitation.

Consequently, any practitioner who expects a passive and totally compliant patient had better avoid those with long-term disability (and some do for this very reason). These survivors insist on making decisions regarding their own bodies and will not automatically comply with recommendations and procedures with which they do not agree. Their social skills have been honed to detect "bullshit" and insincerity, and their survival has depended on this skill.

Over time, as function declines, a certain egocentricity sets in, which is both a product of and a further stimulus to survival. The world may narrow to a repetitive concern about the nuances of body function and an obsessive worry about environmental obstacles and arrangements. While this egocentricity may have high survival value in a physical sense, it places a strain on relationships with family and friends who find, over time, that their needs may less often be satisfied. Thus, this is a further imbalance that must be handled.

During an interview with one couple who has been married over 40 years, the wife expressed resentment that her entire adult life has been spent helping him manage the disability while shouldering a large percentage of the family responsibilities by herself. Now she is aging and wants some time for her own life, yet he needs her more than ever. When I asked him how he felt when he heard such complaints, he acknowledged that they had discussed this before. He said, "I feel badly that it has worked out this way, but these days I've become very egocentric in order to keep on going, and I just don't have the energy to devote to much else." By all evidence, this has been a loving and solid marriage, but such are the issues that arise at this point in their lives.

This introduces the issue of respite care; the opportunity for the person with a disability to receive proper attention while the family member or caregiver takes a break. Rather than an unnecessary luxury, this can be a key feature in maintaining the health and well-being of the care-giver whose own health needs to be protected, not only for humane reasons but to ensure the continuance of low-cost personal care services that only family members give. However, the cost of a week or two in a nursing home is prohibitively expensive, well beyond the financial resources of most families. Consequently, there never is a vacation from the hard work of living with a severe disability for the disabled person and seldom for the family member.

Locus of Control

The concept of locus of control may be central to the overall process of adjusting to disability (Trieschmann, 1980). There are differences among people in the degree to which they believe that they have personal control over rewards. People with an external locus of control believe that rewards and punishments in life occur as the result of fate, luck, and powerful others. Internals, however, believe that their own actions are the key to success or failure. The critical issue is not the reality of or the physical nature of control but the person's learned belief or expectancy about the relationship between his or her behavior and outcomes. Research (Swenson, 1976) has demonstrated that soon after onset of SCI, those with an internal locus of control have fewer medical problems, are more active, productive, and satisfied with life. This was unrelated to severity of disability. Thus, one would hypothesize that individuals with major physical disability who survive successfully for 30 or more years are more likely to have an internal orientation than external. Yet, does locus of control vary over time? How is it influenced by the experience of long-term disability? The people interviewed for this report have predominantly been internals—they have a deep belief in their ability to influence what happens to them. Each of our biographies demonstrates this concept very well. When faced with an environment that said, "No, you can't," they said, "Oh yes, I will."

Now as function declines, the need to remain in charge and the expectation that they can "do" something to make life better is still strong. They are painfully aware that you cannot count on anyone else. As a result, their anxiety rises as they realize that they have less energy to continue to manipulate the environment. Their frustration tolerance is lowering and they become more easily irritated and annoyed, yet they remain committed to the idea that they will be able to make things work out.

There may indeed be some individuals with an external locus of control who survive successfully for 30 or more years with a major physical disability. However, I would predict that these people have an extremely supporting environment and a very strong body with few weak points. It is highly probable that the supportive environment centers on one key individual, a wife or a mother, for example, who has a very strong internal locus of control herself. Even among men with an internal locus of control, it seems fair to hypothesize that their wives are more likely to have an internal orientation than external. All of these are interesting questions for future research.

Schultz and Decker (1984) studied 100 persons with paraplegia and quadriplegia of 20 or more years' duration. This sample included traumatic and nontraumatic onset of disability. Median age was 56, 90% were male, and 72% were married. They found that perceived control over life was correlated with measures of well-being. Crisp (1984) found that those who had been disabled more than 5 years with their spinal injury and had an internal locus of control were more productive than externals. O'Brien (1981) studied the relevance of locus of control to measures of well-being in retired but nondisabled persons. Those with an internal orientation expressed greater satisfaction with retirement and life in general than externals. Number of physical symptoms was not a good predictor of life satisfaction but internal orientation was.

Thus, one can hypothesize that individuals with long-term disability and an internal locus of control will be highly resistant to efforts to reduce their control or to constrict their environmental options. Their very well-being is highly dependent on remaining free to manage their own lives and is probably highly correlated with the will to live. What happens to the mortality rate if these people lose their freedom to control their own lives? Do internals continue to cope with this issue better than externals or do they give in and die sooner? At the end of their lives, does an external orientation allow one to cope better because there was less expectancy of control and therefore less turmoil when control is lost? These will be fruitful areas for research.

Mood

Traditionally, there has been the expectation that people get exceedingly depressed after onset of a disability, but research has demonstrated that this is not true (Trieschmann, 1980; Howell et al., 1981; Richards, 1986). Schultz and Decker (1984) found that those living with a disability of 20 or more years perceived their lives to be as good as those of people in general, and there was evidence of a tendency to see the positive side of life rather than to dwell on the negative. That certainly was obvious in my interviews for this report. While people were frighteningly aware of the potential problems in the future, generally they did not dwell on them and basically tried to take each day at a time. Others have mentioned the importance of minimizing obstacles even though one is aware of their existence. Thus, it is a matter of philosophy and attitude: Is the glass half full or half empty?

In any discussion of emotionality, it is important to pay attention to semantics and the connotation of words so that we do not miscommunicate. The terms "depression" and "denial" have historically been used in the field of psychiatry to describe an abnormal response to life events. Depression is generally characterized by loss of appetite, insomnia, psychomotor retardation, feelings of hopelessness and helplessness, lack of pleasure in anything, and dysphoric mood extending over a period of time. Denial implies the refusal to acknowledge the existence of a situation or event. Both of these terms have been misused and overused in the field of physical disability by professionals who have failed to perceive the tremendous ability to cope of those with major disabilities (Trieschmann, 1980). Goldiamond (1976) addressed this issue very eruditely.

As we deal with people who are aging, it is important that we differentiate between depression and unhappiness and between denial and hope or the determination to overcome obstacles. Nobody that I interviewed was depressed; some were unhappy about immediate problems, and all were concerned about their future ability to remain free and functional. Everyone was going about his or her life with stoicism and determination to be as active and involved in their usual activities as possible. Thus, it will be important to use our terms precisely, and use the term "depression" only when it is strictly appropriate. For example, in the case of a physically disabled person refusing to accept more adaptive equipment when it is recommended by health professionals, it is important to determine whether it is strength and determination or denial that is behind the refusal. In most cases, it probably is the former, since most people are painfully aware of their altered abilities and sensations and do not deny their existence. Rather, the timing may be wrong for the acceptance of more adaptive equipment. Most changes of this nature involve tradeoffs of restrictions of one kind for freedoms of another kind. For example, many are faced with the decision of accepting an electric wheelchair in addition to or instead of a manual one. Although this conserves the person's energy by eliminating the need to push oneself over carpets or rough terrain, it is heavier and cannot fit into a regular automobile. As a result, one must purchase a van with a hydraulic lift, an expensive proposition. Vans get lower gasoline mileage (an additional expense) and may not be as easy to park. Another reason for resisting such equipment is that it emphasizes the image of disability, not an easy thing to take on after fighting to be as "normal" as possible.

Sally and Dave have adopted an electric chair and van without concern for the image of disability because they have limited muscle function available to do the work of the lower half of the body; consequently, exhaustion prevented them from being as active as they would like. Consequently, the van and chair meant less disability to them but tremendously greater expense. For Clifford, however, not walking and accepting a wheelchair meant to him a loss of function and the reality of the disability for the first time. Thus, he resisted it until he had no choice. Bill has accepted crutches and occasional use of a wheelchair with reasonable equanimity because he is aware of the alternative: confinement to bed. Frank and Jack do not have the need for further adaptive equipment yet, and Paul, because of his high level of quadriplegia and age at onset, has had the full package of adaptive equipment since discharge from acute hospitalization.

Any studies on the mood of those with long-term disability should definitely use as a control group those of similar age, with and without medical problems. It will be important to understand and utilize the base rates (average frequency of occurrence) of irritability and unhappiness in older groups in general so as not to overestimate and overinterpret the incidence in those with long-term disability. Furthermore, all of the methodological issues regarding the assessment of emotional and psychological states described by Trieschmann (1980) apply to this current situation as well. Of particular importance is the matter of how mood or emotion is defined and *measured*. The cheap and easy way is to devise a rating scale for the purposes of the research and then have staff or others rate the person on the emotional state being studied. However, without evidence of reliability and *validity*, this is a worthless procedure. It is important to remember that the battlefield of psychology is littered with the bodies of those who underestimated the complexity of this measurement problem. Thus, multidimensional measures, using behavioral, physiological, and ratings by self and others, are the methods of choice (Trieschmann, 1980).

Gender

Aging is a woman's problem: she takes care of others as they grow old and then struggles to take care of herself as she ages alone. It will be extremely relevant to examine the roles that wives and mothers of disabled men play, as well as sisters, nieces, and daughters, but that issue is addressed below under the topic of family and interpersonal support. However, the concept of gender of the disabled person is very relevant when we study the topic of aging.

Within the spinal cord injury population, the current ratio of men to women is 4 to 1 (Young et al., 1982), but it is possible that men outnumber women even more in the older generation of SCIs because of the incidence of SCI in the military. Within the polio group, the number of men and women should be almost equal, but Halstead et al. (1985) found that women responded to their questionnaire in greater numbers than men did. Thus, the actual incidence of men and women who are experiencing aging with disability problems is unknown.

Geisler et al. (1977) reported that women with SCI accounted for 13% of the sample but only 10% of the deaths. Why? In general, women in the United States have a greater life expectancy than men, but does this account for the difference? How do women handle the aging process in comparison to men? Do they have the same types of biological–organic problems and do they have the same emotional responses?

It is probable that a large percentage of women with disabilities will face the aging process alone, either because their husbands died earlier or because they have lived alone for years. Crewe et al. (1979) reported on the marriages and divorces in a civilian SCI population. Five of the six women who were married at injury were later divorced in comparison to six of 29 men. Furthermore, there is reason to believe that women with major disabilities have a lower probability of entering a marriage contract than disabled men. Trieschmann (1980) discusses the social issues of disability and the roles that physical capability and attractiveness play in all social relationships. Within the "nondisabled" group, physical attractiveness seems to be a primary criterion for many men in selecting women with whom to date and relate. As a result, many physically disabled women find that men avoid them because of the disability and seldom take the time to find out who the person really is. Women with disabilities will display the same range of wonderful and lovable features as women without disabilities; they are no better and no worse as partners. Luckily, there are also some men who do not allow physical issues to become paramount.

Thus, what is the impact of this period of aloneness on the process of aging in women? Do women age faster than their disabled male counterparts or does the period alone equip them very well for the struggle to survive as an older person? Many of the men that I interviewed had exceedingly close relationships with their wives and the thought of the wife's death was positively devastating to them. Do these men have fewer skills physically and emotionally to survive alone than an equally disabled woman does or than a disabled man who never married?

On the average, women seem to be better at forming networks of relationships for interpersonal support that goes beyond their relationship with a husband or provides input in the absence of a husband. This is very well described in the hearing-impaired community by Becker (1980). Because deaf individuals are often socially isolated from the hearing community, they develop strong social networks for support throughout their lives. This becomes a particular asset when they grow older and a partner dies. The social network remains a powerful factor in their lives, which modulates the impact of a death or divorce.

Disabled women, however, have been doubly discriminated against by society (Deegan and Brooks, 1985). Their status as a woman and a disabled person has placed them at a disadvantage socially and financially throughout their lives, not only in their ability to earn money but in the allocation of social benefits by the state–federal system. Therefore, many of the women in the older age groups, both disabled and "nondisabled" by the way, will be poorer than their male counterparts, since homemaker, wife, mother, and caretaker of the family have never been defined as legitimate vocations by our society. Please recall that Dave and his wife qualify for an allowance of $700 a month for her services as an attendant to him. If they were not married, they would receive $900 for the same purpose. Consequently, income on which to survive will be a critical issue to evaluate when comparing perception of the aging process among men and women with disabilities.

Thus, do men with disabilities have a higher probability of being taken care of by family when older? Are older disabled women more likely to end up in a nursing home than men? If this is the case, is it lack of financial resources, lack of interpersonal support, or a combination of the two that accounts for the entry into such a facility? Or are women more resourceful at creating environmental supports to stay out of nursing homes than men once their wives can no longer care for them? Obviously, there is a multitude of issues that deserves to be studied in this area.

THE ENVIRONMENTAL (E) IMPACT OF THE AGING PROCESS

Over the life span with a disability, a reasonable balance had been achieved among the P, O, and E variables. The original alteration in the O function, the biological–organic features of the human system, required an accommodation in P and E variables to produce an equilibrium—harmony—adjustment—health, all facets of the same outcome. There was an expenditure of great personal resources, and there was a need to adapt the environment for optimal function. Now with aging, there are additional changes in the biological function that tip the balance, put the system into disharmony, require new adjustments to be made, and could lead to a decline in overall health status unless the P,O,E balance is restored.

In any disabled person's life, the environment (E) really defines the extent and nature of the handicap: the social environment, physical environment, and financial environment. In their earlier years, as our biographies have demonstrated, people who have disabilities but no financial compensation have to expend great personal resources in order to achieve a high enough income to survive comfortably and independently or in order to work the system to barely survive if they cannot earn a high income. They were able to overcome inadequate environmental supports by sheer willpower and determination. However, as the energy to continue the battle declines, reliance on extraordinary will and determination may not be enough. Rather, the role of the environment as an asset or liability becomes paramount in importance. Therefore, we discuss the impact of money, interpersonal support, knowledgable health professionals, community support services, and role models on the process of aging with a disability because it is these factors that determine quantity and quality of life for all older people, disabled and "nondisabled" alike.

The Financial Implications of Aging with a Disability

Living with a disability during one's most vital adult years is expensive; however, the impact of aging is to increase the costs even further while potentially reducing one's ability to earn money to cover these costs if not covered by disability compensation. The increased costs are associated with the purchase of adaptive equipment, the modification of the living environment, the employment of personal care attendants and other services, and the payment of the proportion of medical care not covered by third-party payers.

Most people with major physical disabilities utilize adaptive equipment, crutches, braces, or a wheelchair, to facilitate function. Use of this equipment usually puts a strain on the upper extremities to push the wheelchair, to transfer in and out of the wheelchair, and to get the wheelchair in and out of the back seat of the car. As energy declines and joints, tendons, and muscles protest against such exertions, the person is faced with a choice: reduce the frequency and kind of activities or use other equipment to accomplish the task. Having a choice, however, is dependent on having income or disability benefits to purchase such equipment. A regular wheelchair (manual propulsion and traditional design) costs approximately $1,000, whereas the newly designed lightweight chairs can cost in excess of $1,600. A wheelchair cushion costs $250 and, of course, is a necessity to prevent pressure sores. The electric wheelchair costs approximately $5,000; considerably more, depending on the features an individual might need.

Pulling the chair in and out of the car takes its toll on shoulders and arms; thus, some people use an electric wheelchair lift, which raises the chair into a carrier on top of the car. These very helpful devices cost approximately $2,000. Electric wheelchairs, of course, cannot be placed in the car; they are too heavy to be lifted and do not fold together because of the battery and other apparatus. So purchasing an electric wheelchair also entails the additional expense of purchasing a van with hydraulic lifts, automatic electric doors, and access for the wheelchair at the driver's panel. To spend $20,000–25,000 is not unusual. The lower gasoline mileage of such vehicles increases the cost even more, and in hot areas of the country, extra air conditioning may need to be installed.

The wives or other family members may have helped with transfers in the past or need to do so now that the person is older. But chances are that the wife is older too and may have her own health problems. Therefore, a lift apparatus may take the strain off backs, shoulders, and necks, but such lifts cost $700. If transfer to the toilet is not longer feasible, a portable commode chair can be purchased for $100.

Home modifications are an additional expense as function declines. A step that could be negotiated in a manual wheelchair becomes an obstacle to an electric one, and, consequently, a ramp needs to be built. Transfers into and out of a bathtub become exceedingly difficult and potentially dangerous as energy declines, and as a result bathroom modifications, always an expensive venture, may be considered. A roll-in shower is an ideal choice, but such a modification can easily run into the thousands of dollars.

Purchase of services is always expensive: if you want to save money, do it yourself. However, people with disabilities often cannot do some things for themselves, and, with age, the amount of assistance needed may increase. Let us consider first the costs of a personal care attendant (PCA). Can you imagine paying the minimum wage for personal care services on which your very survival depends? Finding, training, and keeping good PCAs is a strain even before considering the financial costs. Remember that Paul in our biographies requires help four hours a day, seven days a week, which costs $13,200 a year. As Betty gets older or if she should get sick, how much PCA time will he need? If she got really sick, would he have to go to a nursing home for a while? Nursing homes charge $2,000–2,500 a month for uncomplicated ambulatory patients.

As the disabled person and family member get older and less able to do as much, housekeeping, laundry, gardening, and home maintenance services may need to be purchased. Because families are dispersed over a wide geographical area, free assistance from sons and daughters is not always available; thus, one has to pay to get things done. Moving out of a home into a condominium or retirement community may seem to be a good idea, but is it? Many new condominiums are built to minimum standards and are often inaccessible or unsuitable for wheelchair living. Narrow door widths, narrow hallways, and multi-level dwellings are common in many condominiums and therefore are not an option for those with major disabilities. Some of my informants have found that retirement communities are often inaccessible to those in wheelchairs, and, furthermore, some refuse admission to anyone living in a wheelchair, stating that their policy is to accept only those in good health, i.e., walking. No amount of discussion was able to change that policy according to one woman, a widow of 69, who has had a spinal injury for 30 years.

The financial commitments of such retirement communities are often formidable whether disabled or not. Typically, one "purchases" one's unit for $17,000 or more, plus pays a monthly maintenance fee of $500 or more. Meals, help with cleaning, and laundry are additional charges. If one gets sick and needs to move into the nursing home portion of the community, the monthly charges escalate to typical nursing home fees, and one *loses* one's unit and gets none of the original purchase money back. There is no credit toward future expenses from the initial purchase of the unit. Also, most of these retirement communities have a financial and medical evaluation procedure that is designed to screen out anyone who cannot afford to pay such costs until they die. These communities, of course, are businesses, and they do not want anyone who is on or may end up on Medicaid because Medicaid will not pay the fees they charge. It is interesting to note that a fair proportion of these communities are run by our established religious organizations, which often claim tax-exempt status.

The costs of nursing home placement can rapidly lead to poverty for the rest of the family; a recent example occurred in New York where spouses had to sue their disabled husbands in family court for support (*New York Times*, March 6,

1986). Nursing home costs for a disabled person can amount to $45,000 to $64,000 a year. Medicaid is the only public-assistance insurance that pays for this but only after the individual or couple has depleted most of their personal savings, a concept called "spending down." In one recent case in New York, the woman had been a housewife and mother, had taken care of her disabled husband at home for 10 years, but, when she injured herself, at age 75, she was forced to place him in a nursing home. The nursing home charges amounted to $64,000 a year.

The couple rented an apartment, had $22,000 in savings accumulated during 50 years of marriage, and had an income of $1,887 a month (his Social Security and work pension totaled $1,665 and her Social Security contributed $222). Medicaid rules allowed the couple to keep $4,400 in savings, establish a $1,500 burial fund for each, and to keep $424 a month for the wife to live on. The remainder of their savings and monthly income was applied to the cost of the nursing home care. Thus, in effect she was reduced to poverty status after a lifetime of hard work.

It is interesting to note how the rules deal with the spouse's Social Security income in such situations. She was allowed to keep her Social Security stipend of $222 and was given $202 of his Social Security. If their roles had been reversed, however, and she was the disabled person, the state law would permit her husband to keep his Social Security (just like his wife was permitted hers) if he needed this money to live on. Thus, he would have been allowed $1,665 a month (his pension and his Social Security) for living expenses, whereas she was allowed only $424 (her Social Security and only part of his). Is this an example of why some claim that women in fact do not have equal rights under the law?

One could argue that this is not unequal treatment because he was allowed to keep his entire Social Security and, indeed, she was allowed to keep hers. Thus, the issue is, "How much of his Social Security is she entitled to receive?" His is larger because he worked outside of the home, but she worked for 50 years *inside* of the home. Society has not valued women's work as homemakers despite the fact that the estimated costs of such services, if purchased, would amount to over $30,000 a year, suggesting that the current guidelines should be changed to credit the role of homemaker in the economic partnership of marriage. In the case cited above, the wife eventually filed suit in Family Court and was awarded $1,099 a month, twice as much as Medicaid had allowed her.

Good medical care often, but not necessarily always, depends on the ability to pay. Within the civilian sector, the issue revolves around the percentage of costs that the individual pays and the third-party payer pays. Currently, there is increasing pressure to increase the percentage that the individual pays under Medicare and to reduce the number of services covered by Medicare and Medicaid. (Medicare covers a percentage of certain health care costs for those aged 65 and older. Medicaid covers certain health care costs of those earning very low incomes and those on SSDI and SSI.) Those individuals covered by Medicaid often find that many physicians will not accept them as patients because of the low fees paid. Thus, physicians receive counsel in such journals as *Medical Economics* (Rusley, 1984) on how to gear their practice toward first-class or super-saver medicine (those are the terms used in the article). First-class medicine (class 1) is for those patients who put quality, comfort, and convenience above cost considerations (i.e., have insurance and funds to pay beyond insurance coverage), whereas super-saver medicine is geared to those enrolled in health maintenance organizations and similar prepaid plans (class 2) and those covered by Medicaid and Medicare (class 3). For class 2 and 3 patients, physicians are advised that they maximize their income by increasing the volume of patients seen, which requires office assistants, who will help the physician see the maximum number of patients in the minimum amount of time. In dealing with the "first-class" patients, excellence of service is considered to be essential, which includes a high-overhead establishment and large amounts of the physician's personal time. "Your manner throughout must be relaxed and unhurried. On subsequent visits, take the time to familiarize yourself with patients [sic] charts before you meet with them. Primary care practitioners can focus more on 'wellness' programs, perhaps helping people improve their nutrition and exercise programs. And never insist that a class 1 patient pay you at the time of service—you must make it clear that you trust him" (Rusley, 1984, p. 102).

Within the veteran population, most nonservice-connected disabled veterans have little extra income and therefore depend on the VA for care. But many service-connected disabled veterans (who qualify for top priority free care at the VA) do have the income to give them a choice, and 50% of my service-connected informants choose to get care in the civilian sector.

Thus, those who have survived 30 or more years are well tuned to their body's function and try to give it first-class care. However, ability to pay determines whether or not the person will receive first-class treatment, and even service-connected disabled veterans have frequently had trouble getting immediate attention to important problems.

Furthermore, the financial implications of aging with a disability relate not only to additional yearly expenses but also to the reduction in income when one must reduce one's employment, partially or totally. In some families, the "nondisabled" spouse's income is essential to the survival of the couple; therefore, aging and illness of the spouse can be a major financial disaster. Without earned income to supplement the SSDI and Supplemental Security Income benefits, plus the additional expenses outlined above, an independent living situation may no longer be possible. However, our fragmented, poorly coordinated legislation will pay to house someone in a nursing facility but not to keep the person at home.

Interpersonal Support

Living with a major physical disability is hard work for the disabled person and for the family. As a result, the unsung heroines and heroes of any saga of long-term disability are the wives, mothers, and daughters and the husbands, fathers, and sons. Without slighting the contributions of men, it is fair to say that women are more often the caretakers in most families around the world. As a result, aging is a woman's problem: she takes care of others and then often faces aging when she is all alone.

The women who have lived with severely disabled men have shouldered responsibilities often associated with the male role in addition to the traditional woman's activities of housekeeping, child-rearing, and caretaking. For example, they have cut the lawn, taken out the garbage, put in storm windows, shoveled the snow, carried the suitcases when traveling, monitored or performed home and car repair. Often they have also given some degree of personal care to their disabled husband. Male neighbors seldom offered assistance, and women neighbors were sometimes angry at these wives for setting an example that their own "nondisabled" husbands might expect of them. Some of these wives have also held jobs outside of the home in order to add to the family income. In addition, some of these women currently are accepting the additional burden of taking care of their own aging parents either in their own home or in the parents' home. Now these women are in their 50s and 60s, tired and painfully aware of their own mortality. Some of them have arthritic problems, cardiovascular problems, and other health concerns characteristic of older women, and this all occurs when their husband's energy level and biological function are declining. This increases the amount that they have to do if they cannot afford hired help. Some are angry and honest about it; they have never had any time for themselves because they always have had obligations to care for someone else.

It is important to note that these are highly successful marriages (El Ghatit and Hanson, 1975, 1976) based on trust, sharing, loyalty, and love. Many of these women grew up in the 1930s and 1940s when hard work, duty, and responsibility were accepted without question. But one wonders about some of the young men and women raised in the 1960s and 1970s, often called the "feel good and have it all" generation. Will these marriages in which one partner is disabled be as successful?

And what about the offspring of marriages in which one parent is disabled? Will they help? As young adults in their 20s and 30s, the sons and daughters of disabled war veterans and polio survivors are establishing their own careers and families, struggling with mortgages and education expenses for their own children. Most have little money to spare beyond expenses and, as is characteristic of the American public in general, little money in savings. Often, they live in cities other than the one in which their parents live, and visits are annual, at best semi-annual, events. However, these children are as normal and well-adjusted as those raised by "nondisabled" parents (Buck and Hohmann, 1981), and, thus, this pattern of family relationships is characteristic of many across the United States.

Some with disabilities did not marry and either continued to live with families or have lived alone. The parents (particularly the mothers) of sons and daughters with disabilities have had their caretaking responsibilities extended beyond their own expectations, which has sometimes been a burden, sometimes not. But the issue of burden cuts both ways. No matter how loving the family, to be unable to live independently of parents (whether for financial, physical, or intellectual reasons) can be a psychological burden, since one seldom has a chance to develop self-confidence to the fullest extent possible. Some choose to live with their parents without it implying psychological dependency, but the important issue is choice. When wives or parents age, a major crisis is in the making. Not only may the physical environment change (not living at home any longer), but the interpersonal environment may change as those on whom one counted may not be available for physical or emotional support.

There is a vast literature documenting the role of interpersonal relationships in well-being and health, and a review of this literature is beyond the scope of this document. Lynch (1977, 1985) describes the impact of relationships on cardiovascular health; Becker (1980) describes the importance of social support among the hearing impaired; and Schultz and Rau (1985) discuss the role of social support throughout the life course. But what about the well-being of those giving support?

Bishop et at. (1985) studied the morale and family functioning of 178 "nondisabled" couples in their 60s. They found that health status and family functioning have a stronger association with morale than socioeconomic status does, and that husbands and wives differ on these relationships. The husband's morale was most strongly associated with health status, socioeconomic status, and income and to a lesser degree with family functioning, whereas the wife's morale was most strongly associated with family functioning and to a lesser degree health and socioeconomic status. However, these factors accounted for less than one-third of the variance in morale. Clearly, morale is a very complex issue. Whether or not these results would be found in a group in which one partner had been disabled for a long time is not known.

Taking a slightly different approach, Schultz and Wood (1985) interviewed 67 caregivers of persons with paraplegia and quadriplegia (traumatic and nontraumatic origin) to assess factors associated with psychological well-being. They found that high levels of psychological well-being were associated with their own good health, high levels of perceived control, the feeling that they receive adequate social support, and that they are satisfied with the quantity and quality of their social contacts. Social contact with family and friends was extremely important regardless of how supportive such contact was. Depression was correlated with the magnitude of the physical burden and the amount of assistance the disabled person needed.

Consequently, families have played a powerful role in maintaining the well-being of persons with disabilities. The relationship has produced benefits to both parties without a doubt, but the caregiver has carried a burden as well as the person with the disability. As they age, each is experiencing less energy, more biological dysfunction, and, thus, the P,O,E balance for each and for the family unit itself is being challenged. This happens in all families, disabled and "nondisabled," but in the former group, the physical burden on the caregiver has been great and may get greater as their ability to cope with it declines. As a result, interpersonal support for the caregiver is terribly important in these later years. The role of many variables, health of each party, perceived control over life events, amount, type, and quality of social relations and economic security should be evaluated for the disabled person and caregiver separately, since the results seem to vary in each group. The Schultz and Decker (1984) and Schultz and Wood (1985) studies should be expanded to include a group more representative of those with long-term disability (their age range was great) and should include economic status as an independent variable. Caregiver should be defined more uniformly so that we can explore the possible differences when the caregiver is male versus female, husband, son, mother, wife, or daughter. Age and generation of the caregiver may be a factor in these results.

The issue of income and financial security comes up again, especially in the context of interpersonal support, because the family member caregiver may not be as physically able to manage the same range of household responsibilities as previously and may not be able to give added assistance to the disabled person. This worry about money can strongly influence a relationship and the perceived burden of the caregiver. Furthermore, many couples with whom I talked were worried about the wife's widowhood and spent more time explicitly planning for it than others may: What income would she have? Could she afford to keep their home? Since the expenses of mere living were greater throughout their married life, chances are that the surviving, "nondisabled" spouse may have fewer financial resources than average. Any study of this issue should clearly differentiate between service-connected disabled veterans and others.

But what if the nondisabled caregiver, especially a spouse, dies first? What impact will this have on the disabled survivor, emotionally, biologically, and in terms of living circumstances? The base rates of reaction to widow and widower status in the "nondisabled" community should be considered in any research of this issue.

When we look at the issue of policy and research in this area, there are a few core concepts that must be kept in mind. Since the human and the family unit are P,O,E systems, biological–organic changes associated with aging will influence the P and E variables of the disabled individual and of the caregiver. Thus, to focus exclusively on the person with the disability is short-sighted, since the impact of changes in function spreads to family and friends: the caregivers' well-being (P), physical function (O), and resources (E) will influence the well-being and function of the disabled person, and, consequently, a systems approach, a health care approach, is truly appropriate here.

Schultz and Decker (1984) and Shultz and Wood (1985) found that perception of control over one's life is tremendously important to the well-being of both the disabled person and caregiver. This goes back to the concept of locus of control and freedom to make decisions as to how one will live, the latter dependent not only on personal resources but also on environmental resources: money to meet the increased expenses and a system of community support services aimed at keeping people in their own homes. Furthermore, a knowledgable group of health-oriented professionals and facilities is essential to achieving this goal.

Knowledgable Health Professionals and Facilities

In Chapter 3, we discussed the concept of health, aging within the context of health, and the characteristics of a health care system (Table 3-3). As biological–organic (O) changes occur with aging, these changes cannot necessarily be eliminated or cured. In many cases, these changes define a new status of what is, what must be adjusted to; as a result, treatment aimed only at biological–organic variables will be less successful at ameliorating the imbalance in health than interventions directed at the optimal utilization of personal and environmental resources. Therefore, our traditional sickness treatment system and the professionals trained in this approach will misperceive the nature and scope of the problem. Survivors of long-term disability are exceedingly knowledgable of the workings of their bodies but *they desperately need health-oriented professionals to join in partnership with them; professionals who understand the nature of the biological decline; professionals who understand the complexity of the P,O,E balance; and professionals who will suggest interventions aimed at O variables, P variables, and E variables.*

People with long-term SCI and the residuals of polio feel particularly disenfranchised by the medical establishment. We have a series of 13 Model Regional Spinal Cord Injury Treatment Centers nationally that were mandated to provide a system of services to those with spinal cord injury. This system was to include the coordination of proper emergency medical services at the scene of the accident and in the hospital, acute medical management and rehabilitation, outpatient services designed to foster the opportunity for a full life, and long-term follow-up. However, in effect, most of the centers allocate the majority of their resources to coordination of emergency medical services with acute rehabilitation care for newly injured SCIs. Long-term disability within such a context is 18–60 months after injury. Research and clinical services are focused primarily on helping people get established in the first months and years after injury, but few have planned any services to meet the needs of long-term SCI. They are charged with the responsibility to follow up those treated acutely at their centers, but the longest duration is now 13 years. Unfortunately, 44.6% of the cases at some centers have been lost to follow-up over a 10-year period. These centers have not taken deliberate steps to make themselves known to those with long-term SCI in the community or in their region, and they have not been particularly effective at educating the regional medical establishment about management of long-term SCI problems. In truth, these centers have not given a great deal of thought to those with long-term disability who were not seen for the acute injury at their center.

Within the VA, many hospitals without SCI centers are not enthusiastic about treating people with long-term physical disabilities. One of my inform-ants who has a service-connected disability of 40 years' duration reports that, when he is admitted for treatment of a medical problem, quite frequently he will be discharged dangerously early from his local VA because the staff not only has no knowledge of his disability problems but seem frightened of them. He is not a hypochondriac but a highly successful and independent person who happens to be very capable of assessing the quality of medical interven-tion that he receives. Therefore, he often seeks medical care within the civilian community, paid for out of his own pocket, and looks forward to the day when he qualifies for Medicare.

The stories about experiences with the VA SCI centers vary, not so much by person as by center. Some centers are perceived as good and caring, particu-larly because of a few key professionals who provide leadership and personal regard for the human being involved. Other centers are viewed as mixed bless-ings: an individual may receive free care but at a personal and occasionally a physical cost. There are many stories from my informants about unsupervised medical residents who barely conceal their distaste for their current clinical assignment, who view those rows of disabled people in bed as barely human, and who tend to view their rotation as an opportunity to experiment.

The admission procedures at some VAs and SCI centers have been described as monuments to bureaucratic ineptitude and heartlessness. One wife told me of sitting with her husband for eight hours in the admissions waiting room while he was in severe pain without any medical attention. At 4:30 p.m., the clerks closed the office and told them to come back the next day. When the wife protested that they had driven over 50 miles to get there, they were told to get a motel room for the night. He is service-connected and therefore receives "top priority" for admission. Another informant who has been living with his SCI for 35 years reports that it often takes two to three weeks for urine cultures to be processed at his VA outpatient urology clinic. By the time that medication is prescribed by the physician, a raging infection is in progress, which takes even longer to heal. Is this good medical management?

As a person ages, a variety of body systems may be the scene of difficulty, not only those body systems associated with the disability. Thus, some of my informants have expressed concern over the lack of program managership on the part of a physician who knows about the disability but who can also inte-grate the treatments recommended for other biological problems into an over-all plan of living with the disability. Several different specialists, each expert in certain body systems, may make recommendations without any one person assessing the overall impact of these interventions or the potential interactive side-effects. Who is paying attention to the potential impact of a medication to treat a cardiovascular problem on already compromised kidney function?

One individual, service-connected, who lives 30 minutes from a major VA SCI center fears that in a medical emergency he may die if taken to the VA hospital because of the delays and bureaucratic procedures involved with transportation to the hospital and admission. As a result, he has given instructions to his family to take him to the emergency room of a civilian hospital an equal distance away even though he'd have to pay for the care himself. Although the hospital really does not know much about physical disability problems per se, emergency medical management is more promptly available. "You know, I've come to the conclusion that after all of these years of surviving relatively well with the disability, I may die because the system is just not set up to deal with my type of problems."

All of my informants have talked about the number of wonderful, caring, and dedicated people who work at the VA hospitals. However, one major problem is the number of employees who do not care about the patient as a human being. These latter types seem to see the civil service system as a guaranteed annual income until they qualify for federal retirement benefits. People are not easily fired for nonperformance and these individuals stay and create a most unhealthy climate. Unfortunately, those in this category can be found in all job assignments from physicians down to the lowest paid person. Consequently, the issue is not one of education or professional role but a system in which no effective negative consequences are attached to mediocre or bad performance.

Now the other side of the picture must be stated. What about the highly dedicated and caring people who strive to give good care within such a climate? They do their best often against great odds. One wonderful physican described his concerns and difficulties in providing good medical management to 160 patients with only three full-time physicians. The rules state that they are not to work more than 40 hours a week without reimbursement for overtime, but there is no money for overtime. When a physician is sick or away at a conference, two people cover 80 patients each. If evening or weekend emergencies occur requiring the physicians' presence, their daytime hours should be reduced accordingly so that the total is not more than 40 hours for the week. My informant ignores the rules for himself, works 12 hours a day, and does the best that he can do to bring good care to his friends with SCI, and thus is perceived as a good man by all with whom I talked. There are equally dedicated individuals in all positions at all VAs, but the overall *system* for delivery of care is seriously flawed.

In asking for suggestions to remedy these problems, no one proposed that we eliminate the VA hospital system. Many wanted the choice to use the civilian sector if they wanted, the care to be reimbursed by the VA. Some wanted to receive all of their treatment at their VA SCI center despite the problems because of the social network among the long-term SCIs who all receive treatment there. Admission to the hospital usually will provide the opportunity to see old friends, which helps to modulate the concern about the bureaucracy and the care. There is no question but that the VA system is loyally supported by a significant percentage of veterans, but all believe that there is room for significant improvement in efficiency of procedures and quality of personnel. *Unfortunately, further budget cuts without improvement in efficiency of procedures and quality of personnel may increase total national costs ultimately, not reduce them.* In the short term, money may be saved by eliminating certain services and personnel, but in the long term, such reductions may lead to very expensive medical complications that would have been prevented in a full-service system.

With an aging veteran population, a significant proportion of whom are disabled, a fragmented sickness treatment approach will underestimate the complexity of the aging problem, will apply intermittent biologically oriented (O) treatments, and will ignore the psychosocial (P) and environmental (E) factors in the human equation. Budget cuts are usually aimed at the virtual elimination of psychosocial and environmental services to the disabled and the reduction of access to biological–organic treatments. Unfortunately, this is a prescription for disaster. *Rather than a reduction of services, there needs to be a complete reassessment of the service delivery system so that the funds allocated are effectively directed to reducing the health problems of this population, thereby reducing the need for further costly services.* While this is a potentially incendiary topic, the need to cut the federal deficit can be an opportunity to make changes that improve our approach to long-term disability rather than merely to reduce services. This latter approach essentially means disenfranchising one group in favor of another, i.e., rationing of health care. Surely an advanced civilization such as ours can find a better approach than this.

In many ways, it is a subgroup of the polio survivors who seem to be experiencing some of the most dramatic biological–organic (O) changes that are having a devastating impact on psychosocial (P) and environmental (E) issues in their lives. For example, one woman in her early 40s, wife, mother, and career woman who walked with only a limp, found that her energy level and muscle function declined rapidly over a one-year period. Her physician advised her to quit her job, stay home, use a wheelchair, and be up no more than a couple of hours at a time. She had been athletic, active, and involved in a variety of community events. This is, in some ways, the sudden onset of a new disability (new in dimension and implications), which will entail all of the psychosocial adjustment issues described by Trieschmann (1980). How does this woman adjust to inactivity after a lifetime of activity? What activities does she use to fill her days productively in order to avoid depression and to remain healthy? How does this influence her relationship with her teenage children and husband? What pressures and emotions does the husband experience as he struggles to remain sympathetic despite losing his companion for many of their mutually rewarding activities and interests? Consequently, to treat only the energy level and muscle function without regard for the massive changes in lifestyle is foolish.

While physicians certainly understand the implications of such a change in function, they are not trained to deal with these issues, and our sickness treatment approach does not have a coordinated package of services to assist people in making adjustments of this kind. Thus, the physician might recommend counseling by a psychologist to help her cope with her feelings about her new situation. But that is not sufficient. These are reality problems about which one has a legitimate series of emotions, and, thus, counseling by a psychologist within the context of a full-spectrum rehabilitation program is the intervention of choice. How can her environment be arranged to facilitate rewarding function without encouraging further physical decline? How can we help the family unit to work together so that a schism does not develop to isolate her from family events? Thus, we need a program to deal not only with the feelings but the loss of valued activities, a program that assists the person to find meaning in life, reasons for getting out of bed in the morning.

The American Association of Medical Colleges (1984) has recently issued a report that recommends changes in medical education aimed at increasing the interpersonal and clinical relevance of material taught. That is a worthy start. In addition, rehabilitation specialists should disseminate information in the journals of the individual medical specialties (neurology, orthopedics, pulmonary, internal medicine, urology, family practice) to broaden the outlook of individuals in these fields. Furthermore, disability and aging clinics should be organized to offer the spectrum of health professionals and services needed to provide proper assistance to persons experiencing a decline. But without a doubt, at a policy level, we need to reduce the fragmentation in our social legislation and to re-orient the system so that it is easier to keep people in their own home rather than to send them to a nursing home.

Community Support Services

When one's scope of activities becomes limited, outside assistance for personal care may be required. Assistance with bathing, grooming, dressing, bladder and bowel care and with homemaking activities may make the crucial difference between staying in one's home or not. However, locating and training such a person is not easy and the costs become significant. Paul and Betty, in one of our biographies, have the luxury of coverage by Worker's Compensation and, thus, can pay a wage that gives them high-quality and reliable help. They currently pay $8 an hour to a woman who works 20 hours weekdays and to another person who works eight hours on weekends. Thus, they pay $992 a month for help. Finding help on weekends is not easy, and often people expect a higher rate. PCAs can be obtained through nursing services, the charge ranging from $7–9 an hour. However, people on limited incomes cannot afford such hourly charges and often must rely on those willing to work for $4 an hour, which unfortunately often means a great turnover in personnel. Most people who are really good take a job for this wage only until they can find higher-paying employment.

Some independent living centers (ILCs) have developed a registry of PCAs.

However, there is great variability across ILCs as to whether they thoroughly screen out unsuitable people and whether they provide training.

Therefore, with PCAs there are several issues that need consideration. Among these are the cost or ability to pay for such care; the means by which one locates a PCA; the training the PCA receives; the screening out of psychologically unsuitable people; and the availability of a registry of short-term or emergency help. We have no system, no organization that deals with these issues; rather, each individual requiring help becomes an independent entrepreneur in trying to arrange a workable situation that meets his or her needs. Not only is this an added stress or burden on an already stressed individual, but it is inefficient and may be more costly in the long run. It is probable that on many occasions, people have acquired medical problems because of lack of proper care, which resulted in either costly hospitalization or residence in a nuring home, often at the taxpayer's expense. Does it not make sense for PCA agencies to be developed to meet these needs at a reasonable cost?

The ILC concept has been a worthwhile innovation in the field of rehabilitation and is a result of the social activism of those with physical disabilities in the 1970s. These centers, financed initially through federal money, are resource centers staffed by people with disabilities. Each ILC has the opportunity to develop its own program of services, but peer counseling, advocacy, PCA registry and/or training, directories of accessible housing, and assistance in obtaining adaptive equipment are among the services offered. While there may be variability in the effectiveness of individual ILCs, this concept is a core feature of a true health care system and should be supported as a resource to older disabled individuals.

Home health services are an additional feature of a health care system that is designed to keep people functional and healthy in their homes rather than residing in a nursing home. Such services usually require more professional input and are directed at treating problems that neither require hospitalization nor a skilled nursing facility.

Meal services have been developed that deliver to the person one or two meals daily as needed. These very nicely bridge the gap between having hired help to cook or having to get meals outside of the home.

But when independent living is no longer feasible for either financial or environmental support reasons, what alternatives does a person have? Many retirement homes are not available to people with physical disabilities, either because of high cost or because they discriminate against the handicapped. Such discrimination can take the form of designing and building units with sufficient architectural barriers so that elimination of those with disabilities is built right into the system, so to speak. A skilled nursing facility, i.e., nursing home, is often the only alternative even though the person does not need skilled nursing. Actually, a large percentage of residents of these facilities do not need skilled nursing (Kayser-Jones, 1981). Rather, they are old and need supervised living or physical assistance—but not nursing. Yet, we warehouse our older people in settings that are programmatically designed to reduce function, not maintain it. Certainly, there are recreation programs and social programs but these are frosting on an inedible cake; the person is neither encouraged to nor allowed to participate in daily survival activities of cooking, cleaning, maintenance, gardening, etc. These services are provided and paid for in the daily rate, at a high financial cost and at a high psychosocial cost. While being at home often is lonely and stressful, it does keep people active and fully alive. The body and mind respond to challenge; they decline in the absence of demand.

We have a certain number of severely disabled people who have resided in hospitals or skilled nursing facilities for most of their lives since onset of the disability, not always because they needed skilled nursing but because their home environment could not provide the proper support. In the VA, some individuals with SCI never left the hospital because they did not have the resources to live independently. Some civilians transfer from acute rehabilitation directly to a nursing home because of lack of alternatives in the community. Currently, there is an increasing population of individuals who have survived the original illness or injury but must rely on a respirator for breathing.

Thus, there should be a variety of intermediate steps between totally independent living and skilled nursing facilities. One option is cooperative living. This need not mean segregated living or ghetto-like arrangements. Rather, it is the concept of *shared use of support services all under one roof or dispersed within a neighborhood*. For example, Stock and Cole (1977) studied alternative living environments for those with physical disabilities. Individuals had their own quarters but shared PCAs and other services and were essentially in charge of their own lives. The cost of such living arrangements was significantly less than for a skilled nursing facility.

DeJong (1984) describes the network of alternative living situations for the physically disabled in The Netherlands. Some facilities are large residential units in which hundreds of people live, some are smaller condominium-like facilities, and some are independent apartments in a community linked to a pool of PCAs that are available on call as needed. These living arrangements tend to be systems of services coordinated through government social agencies. The person remains in complete charge of his or her life and contracts for the services needed. There is single-source, single-entry funding for these programs in contrast to our patchwork quilt of social legislation in the United States.

While these services are tied into a slightly different culture and there are some problems that remain unsolved, nevertheless there are some concepts that could be very helpful to the United States as we plan for an aging population. Certainly, a sign of our economic success is the rising proportion of individuals who live into their 70s, 80s, and 90s. Surely such a wealthy country as ours can devote a certain proportion of its gross national product to provide supports to those who helped to create this wealth.

Several features of The Netherlands' program deserve attention. A key to the success of their program is a system of centralized PCAs and clustered housing. With a pool of PCAs available for a certain geographical area, the disabled person can have control over his or her life but access to environmental supports as needed. Essential to the success of this system is that the role of a PCA is considered to be a legitimate occupation with a reasonable wage and certain employment benefits. This creates an atmosphere in which both PCA and disabled person can view the partnership as one that is valuable to each. By pooling resources, PCAs can be paid more, leading to less turnover and a consistently higher caliber of personnel. The single-source financing of all benefits and services eliminates the chronic anxiety that our disabled people experience in the process of discovering programs that will provide assistance and then going through the lengthy application and review processes. Often, our progams stipulate that eligibility for one service precludes eligibility for another, and, thus, single-source financing seems like a veritable paradise in comparison to our current procedures. The Netherlands, years ago, built large residential centers for people with disabilities but over time this concept of segregated living is being rejected as inconsistent with high-quality long-term living. Rather, the current model is clustered housing; a certain percentage of the housing units in certain areas are designed for wheelchair living and the central PCA facility is located nearby. Consequently, *the disabled person is integrated into a normal community neighborhood that is much more acceptable in the long run.*

A final feature of The Netherlands' system deserves attention: disabled persons and providers of services to these persons are both represented on boards and organized into umbrella organizations that devise policy for service delivery. These organizations report to government decision-making bodies that determine the nature of and funding of social programs. Here in the United States, the consumers of health and disability services have never been allowed to play a role in the decision-making process. In addition, various disability groups there have put aside their competitiveness and have joined together to work for the benefit of all.

However, in the United States, the individual is expected to be an entrepreneur from birth to death. We do not make allowances for those whose range of options has been limited by major illness or injury. That seems to be viewed merely as bad luck and a wonderful opportunity to demonstrate whether or not you have the right stuff. Furthermore, we attach great prestige and glamour, devote great sums of money to saving people's lives, but there is little prestige, glamour, or money attached to helping people live, not only exist, after the medical emergency is over. Certainly, in our society, most people would prefer to be free agents who have the opportunity to arrange their lives as they choose. The people with whom I have talked are not asking to be taken care of; they do not seek to avoid responsibility for their own lives; they are not asking for a "handout." Rather, *they request that a system of community support services be available to them in order to be able to remain free and independent. They do not want money to be allocated for bricks and mortar to warehouse them. Rather, they want to remain a part of their own community, with their own friends, their neighbors, their pets and gardens, their furnishings, and all the features that give individuality and character to all of our lives.*

Role Models

In any of our lives, it is helpful to have the opportunity to meet and relate to people who are in comparable situations as we are. We can learn from each other through the sharing of similar experiences as happened, for example, with our World War II SCI veterans. Sometimes, when our mood is at its lowest, the exchange of information with, or introduction to, someone who has experienced and resolved similar problems can be the stimulus for further efforts to overcome current obstacles.

This concept gained great favor in the 1970s as represented by the peer counseling programs within the independent living movement. For newly disabled people, this can be a powerful factor in successfully establishing a new life. However, even for the person who has been disabled for a long time, role models, peer counseling, and support groups can play an important role in maintaining morale and in learning from the experiences of others.

Since we have considered certain disabilities to be static, i.e., SCI, polio, cerebral palsy, spina bifida, etc., a progressive component was not anticipated. Now people are experiencing changes in their lives, and it is reassuring to realize that others are experiencing them too. Many people report that their physicians have told them that self-perceived changes were all in their head and that there was nothing really wrong with them. Thus, support groups often are the only support until the rest of the community becomes more knowledgable about such changes.

However, even when receiving knowledgable and caring input from professionals, there is a lot to be learned from those experiencing the same situation. As a result, support groups and role models will always be a helpful component in a health care system.

THE ADJUSTMENT PROCESS

In all of our lives, aging is synonymous with living. In the lives of those with disabilities, aging is certainly that, but it is also a part of the continual process of adjusting to a disability that resulted from a major illness or injury years ago. All of us are P,O,E systems, and the process of adjustment to the disability involves the struggle to achieve a balance among these influences after a dramatic change in the biological–organic (O) influences in the system. The person (P) comes to terms with the disability and arranges the environment (E), which permits maximum function. Nothing remains the same in any of our lives; there is always change. But the changes in biological–organic (O) function over time may have a greater impact on those with disabilities because it increases the financial, physical, and emotional penalty imposed by the disability.

In this book, we have tried to describe the nature of that penalty and now we must consider what steps we must take as policymakers, as researchers, as teachers, as clinicians, and as individuals to reduce the penalty of disability and the penalty of aging with a disability.

6

Implications for Research and Policy

THE INEQUITIES OF THE SOCIAL WELFARE SYSTEM

The eight individuals presented in our biographies were chosen to represent the variety of environmental circumstances that people with disabilities face. Each individual displayed great strength, fortitude, and resourcefulness to carve out a life that has to be described as "successful adjustment to disability." Each was faced with a physical and financial penalty imposed by the disability, but there were different environmental resources available to each. All used tremendous personal resources to work with the environment and around that environment, but because of inequities in our social legislation, some have had to struggle daily just to survive. Our social legislation reflects the entrepreneurial spirit that has made America great, but it also reflects a callousness, a Darwinian philosophy of survival of the fittest. The disability, however, is a penalty, a handicap, in the great game of survival, and through compensation payments we have partially altered the nature of the handicap for some and not for others. This may be understandable in terms of how our political and legislative system operates, but it is hardly justifiable in a country founded on the principles of justice and democracy.

Depending on your point of view, it is either madness or wisdom to suggest an increase in our social welfare benefits to people with disabilities when the federal budget deficit has reached staggering proportions. It is madness if you view the problem of disability and aging in a fractionated and short-term manner. However, it is wisdom if you view the problem from a systems and long-term point of view. Our social welfare system, through Medicaid, will pay for nursing home placement but will not provide the same (and often less) funds for services that would allow a person to maintain an independent or cooperative living situation. It is highly probable that funds allocated for the latter will be less costly in the short term and long term, so that such a proposal does not represent an actual increase in total national monies allocated to persons with disabilities. This is a proposal to reallocate the funds already being spent to different categories. A single-entry social welfare system with all benefits coordinated through one office should be more cost-effective in the long run rather than the fractionated, crisis-oriented system currently in place. Furthermore, there would be considerable savings in reduced administrative costs alone by eliminating the multiple bureaucracies that are associated with each of our social programs.

Consequently, I would recommend that a bipartisan federal panel be commissioned to study this issue and make recommendations to the President and Congress on changes in our benefits program for those with disabilities. In order to succeed in this task, at least 50% of the commission members should have a major physical or sensory disability or be a family member of someone with cognitive or emotional impairments. In order for this panel to accomplish anything meaningful, *groups with disabilities will have to unify toward a common goal and stop competing against each other*, which only results in benefits for one group reducing the benefits to another group. Civilians and veterans should be on this panel as well as professionals, policymakers, and businessmen. Recommendations of such a commission should have broad implications for research and policy that apply to all aging citizens whether disabled or "nondisabled."

Every day, federal and state treasuries dispense a tremendous amount of money in entitlement payments. To merely reduce the totals spent will not solve the problem of escalating costs. Rather, the tightening of the lid on the federal honey pot is a wonderful opportunity to examine the system and make whatever revisions are necessary to have both a humane and cost-effective social welfare system.

THE TREATMENT APPROACH TO AGING

Since aging is a natural and inevitable part of living, it is reasonable to ask whether aging per se is a problem. Perhaps not (although we usually do not face such a prospect with enthusiasm). Rather, the problem of aging may be in how we define it and how we treat it. Aging has been viewed by some in the traditional medical establishment in terms of diseases and sicknesses that must be analyzed into their component parts through research so that treatments can be identified. But aging is an evolutionary characteristic of a system and therefore needs to be considered as more than biological dysfunction or decline.

A sickness treatment business establishment oriented to acute treatment of biological–organic dysfunctions is the wrong approach, not only to the issue of aging but to the issue of disability. Our society attributes glamour, prestige, and fame to those involved in the saving of lives but denies status and funds to those who work with the ones who have been saved. A health care system guided by a coherent philosophy of the human as a P,O,E system is more suitable to treat most health problems, but particularly those of aging and disability. The field of medical rehabilitation was established on this very premise but unfortunately has not been as successful as hoped at demonstrating a viable alternative to the traditional sickness treatment model. Implicitly rehabilitation believes in the whole person, the importance of the environment, and the need to use a systems approach. However, since an explicit philosophy has never been stated and agreed on by the rehabilitation community, we have been unable to test this model for utility, and we have not noticed how subtly our operational strategies have begun to emulate the traditional model of treatment. If we had explicitly stated our philosophy and tested it, the field of rehabilitation medicine would be in a much stronger position today to demonstrate the cost-effectiveness of rehabilitating those with disabilities and those who are aging with a disability.

A fairly consistent message from all disabled persons is the lack of a true systems approach to long-term problems. This complaint applies to the civilian and VA treatment systems and becomes an indictment of the sickness treatment model of care. Consequently, we need to research and demonstrate a variety of alternatives of health care services that explicitly operate on the philosophy of the human as a P,O,E system. Home health care, ILCs, respite care, pooled PCA services, and cooperative living ventures are all facets of a health care system that needs to be available to disabled and aging persons. How these and other strategies can be used to assist people to remain independent should be a top priority for future research.

THE P,O,E SYSTEM

Our review of the literature on the topic of aging and disability reveals that there are tremendous gaps in our knowledge of the incidence of aging problems and the nature of the problems experienced by those with long-term disability. Much of the research up to now has focused on the question of how long people live after onset of disability and the primary diagnosis at death. However, there are a multitude of other questions more relevant to the lives of those currently living with a major physical disability that remain unanswered.

A top priority for research is a survey of a representative cross-section of the spinal-injured and post-polio populations to determine their functional status at various decades after onset of disability. All of the methodological issues discussed in Chapter 4 must be kept in mind when designing such studies. We need to assess the incidence of various kinds of biological–organic (O) dysfunctions in comparison to a matched group of "nondisabled" individuals in order to determine if the rate and the format of the aging process are influenced by the presence of a major physical disability. Comparisons between the spinal-injured and post-polio groups will help to clarify the issue of format of aging with a disability. It is essential that these incidence surveys utilize samples of people out in the community, not only those seeking treatment for medical problems.

Once we have assessed the range and incidence of biological–organic problems, we can take steps to assess the impact of these biological problems on the person (P) experiencing them and on the environment (E). The reactions of families and spouses should be one focus of such research as well as innovative research and demonstration projects of how to maintain the family as a viable and functional unit.

When the range and incidence of difficulties have been assessed, we will need a series of studies to determine how to prevent, treat, and ameliorate these difficulties. Studies by era of acute management will give indirect information on the prevention of some problems, probably of the genitourinary system in spinal injury, for example. Studies of the role of nutrition, exercise, stress management, and other lifestyle issues will be particularly relevant to the issue of prevention.

In order to assess the role of various P, O, and E variables in survival with a major disability, it would be exceedingly interesting to examine the records of those who died during successive decades after onset to determine if there is a combination of variables that differentiates survivors from those who succumb. The history of rehabilitation is filled with studies that have attempted to predict who will succeed after onset of a disability, with varying results. Possibly it is easier to predict who will not succeed than who will, and it is even possible that we may never be able to predict this issue at all. Perhaps there is no one pattern for success, but many different ones given all the possible combinations and permutations of the P,O,E equation. Furthermore, it is possible that not all of these factors have equal weight, but rather that some have a more powerful influence in certain combinations and a less powerful influence in other combinations. Nevertheless, we have currently among us the ultimate criterion group for such studies.

Certainly, we need to study the incidence, prevention, and treatment of biological–organic dysfunctions in those with long-term disability. But of equal importance are research and demonstration projects of environmental support systems that address the issues discussed in Chapter 5. We need to examine a variety of living arrangements as alternatives to nursing homes. We need to study a variety of solutions to the PCA problem, including the sharing of PCAs. Respite care alternatives need to be assessed in order to keep families from "burning out." Specific support services to the family or spouse need to be researched because they become equal partners in the disability process with increasing age. What types of packages of community support services can be devised to keep people out of nursing homes unless they need skilled nursing services?

Within our current research system, the Veterans Administration has established a series of Geriatric Research, Education, and Clinical Centers (GRECCs) to focus on the problems of an aging veteran population. It seems reasonable to envision that a GRECC devoted to the concept of aging with a physical disability, such a spinal injury, would have utility as a focal point and resource center for research, education, and clinical management of this problem.

The National Institute of Handicapped Research has a series of Rehabilitation Research and Training Centers (RTCs) and Model Regional Spinal Cord Injury Treatment Centers, but none of these centers are specifically focused on the topic of aging with a long-term physical disability. Even though the issue of aging is being generically addressed by two of the RTCs currently, more focused research on this topic would be helpful to our pioneer disabled group. A few of the Model Regional Spinal Injury Centers have initiated some individual research projects directed at the long-term aging disabled population, but the bulk of the resource allocation within these centers is directed at the acutely injured individual.

Even while research is being conducted to assess the incidence of aging problems, there are many projects that could be conducted to enhance the information base of the community family practitioner, internist, and emergency medicine specialist regarding the types of emergencies that seem to be occurring. Information on management of autonomic dysreflexia and urological crises would be a good start, but more effective information dissemination strategies regarding general rehabilitation issues need to be devised.

Research and demonstration projects on alternative methods of health care delivery that demonstrate and test a true health care model should be considered. Contrasting the outcomes of such projects with that of the traditional sickness treatment model would have great utility not only for the disabled but for all individuals with health problems. Such systems would have an outpatient focus, home health focus, in addition to quick and reliable evaluation and treatment of the more frequent biological disturbances (i.e., urological, musculoskeletal, and respiratory) that do not require hospital admission. The human as a P,O,E system should be central to such projects.

THE HUMAN SYSTEM

A basic premise of this book is that the human being is an assemblage or combination of parts that forms a complex and unitary whole. All of us are P,O,E systems, whether disabled or "nondisabled;" if disabled, the disability is only one parameter of the system. Only for discussion purposes can we isolate one parameter from another; but even in the most precisely controlled research it is a fallacy to think that we can truly study one feature of the human system in isolation from the others. That is why we study an event in many people, why we report group averages, and why we use statistical techniques based on the laws of probability. Even quantum physics has recently realized that these laws of probability apply to events in the "hard" sciences.

Soon after onset of a disability, it is possible that a larger number of psychosocial (P) and environmental (E) factors influences one's ability to establish a satisfactory life (Trieschmann, 1974, 1980, 1984b). But as one ages, it is possible that fewer P and E variables influence function. Certainly, the most outstanding of these have been discussed in this book; of course, future research may demonstrate that there are others.

The environment has always been a powerful influence on the quality and even quantity of life for those with disabilities. In the younger years, certain individuals are able to muster great personal resources (P) to overcome environmental (E) obstacles and to succeed despite overwhelming odds. But in the later years of life, one's energy declines and one becomes more vulnerable to the impact of the environment. As a result, any approach to aging (through research or public policy) that focuses primarily on biological–organic (O) issues and that slights the personal (P) and environmental (E) issues is doomed to failure. Consequently, the implications for the future are both fearful and exciting. At a time when we need to reduce massive federal deficits, we have a wonderful opportunity to reassess our strategies for dealing with people who are ill or aging and to transform our system from treating only sickness to promoting health and caring. The latter need not take any more money than the former.

References

Aging America: Trends and projections. U.S. Senate Special Committee on Aging in conjunction with the American Association of Retired Persons, 1984.

Aljure J, Eltorai I, Bradley W, Lin J, Johnson B. Carpal tunnel syndrome in paraplegic patients. *Paraplegia* 1985;23:182–6.

American Association of Medical Colleges. *J Med Educ* 1984;59:1–27.

Barton C, Vaziri N, Gordon S, Eltorai I. Endocrine pathology in spinal cord injured patients on maintenance dialysis. *Paraplegia* 1984a;22:7–16.

Barton C, Vaziri N, Gordon S, Tilles S. Renal pathology in end-stage renal disease associated with paraplegia. *Paraplegia* 1984b;22:31–41.

Becker G. *Growing old in silence.* Berkeley: University of California Press, 1980.

Bishop D, Epstein N, Baldwin L, Miller I, Keitner G. Older couples. I: Morale and family functioning. Unpublished manuscript, Butler Hospital, Providence, RI, 1985.

Blocker W, Merrill J, Krebs M, Cardus D, Ostermann H. An electrocardiographic survey of patients with chronic spinal cord injury. *Am Correct Ther J* 1983;37:101–4.

Blumenthal HT (ed). *Handbook of diseases of aging.* New York: Van Nostrand Reinhold and Company, 1983.

Broecker B, Klein F, Hackler R. Cancer of the bladder in spinal cord injury patients. *J Urol* 1981;125:196–7.

Buck F, Hohmann G. Personality, behavior, values and family relations of children of fathers with spinal cord injury. *Arch Phys Med Rehabil* 1981;62:432–8.

Califano JA Jr. *America's health care revolution.* New York: Random House, 1986.

Capra F. *The turning point: science, society, and the rising culture.* Toronto: Bantam Books, 1982.

Carroll D (ed). History of treatment of spinal cord injuries. *MD State Med J* 1970;19: 109–12.

Cassell E. *The healer's art.* New York: Penguin Books, 1976.

Claus-Walker J, Halstead L. Metabolic and endocrine changes in spinal cord injury: I. The nervous system before and after transection of the spinal cord. *Arch Phys Med Rehabil* 1981;62:595–601.

Claus-Walker J, Halstead L. Metabolic and endocrine changes in spinal cord injury: II (Section 1). Consequences of partial decentralization of the autonomic nervous system. *Arch Phys Med Rehabil* 1982a;63:569–75.

Claus-Walker J, Halstead L. Metabolic and endocrine changes in spinal cord injury: II (Section 2). Partial decentralization of the autonomic nervous system. *Arch Phys Med Rehabil* 1982b;63:576–80.

Claus-Walker J, Halstead L. Metabolic and endocrine changes in spinal cord injury: III. Less quanta of sensory input plus bedrest and illness. *Arch Phys Med Rehabil* 1982c; 63:628–31.

Claus-Walker J, Halstead L. Metabolic and endocrine changes in spinal cord injury: IV. Compounded neurologic dysfunction. *Arch Phys Med Rehabil* 1982d;63:632–8.

Cousins N. *Anatomy of an illness: as perceived by the patient.* New York: W.W. Norton and Company, 1979.

Cousins N. *The healing heart.* New York: Avon Books, 1983.

Crewe N, Athelstan G, Krumberger J. Spinal cord injury: a comparison of preinjury and postinjury marriages. *Arch Phys Med Rehabil* 1979;60:252–6.

Crisp R. Locus of control as a predictor of adjustment to spinal injury. Paper presented at Australian Psychological Society, August 1984.

Dalakas M, Sever J, Fletcher M, Madden D, Papadopoulos N, Cunningham G, Albrecht P. Neuromuscular symptoms in patients with old poliomyelitis: clinical, virological, and immunological studies. In: Halstead L, Wiechers D, eds. *Late effects of poliomyelitis.* Miami: Symposia Foundation, 1985:73–90.

Dalakas M, Elder G, Hallett M, Ravits J, Baker M, Papadopoulos N, Albrecht P, Sever J. A long-term follow-up study of patients with post-poliomyelitis neuromuscular symptoms. *N Engl J Med* 1986;314:959–63.

Deegan M, Brooks N (eds). *Women and disability: the double handicap.* New Brunswick, NJ: Transaction Books, 1985.

DeJong G. *Independent living and disability policy in The Netherlands: three models of residential care and independent living.* New York: World Rehabilitation Fund, 1984.

Dietrick R, Russi S. Tabulation and review of autopsy findings in fifty-five paraplegics. *JAMA* 1958;166:41–4.

El Ghatit A, Hanson R. Outcome of marriages existing at the time of a male's spinal cord injury. *J Chronic Dis* 1975;28:383–8.

El Ghatit A, Hanson R. Marriage and divorce after spinal cord injury. *Arch Phys Med Rehabil* 1976;57:470–2.

El-Masri W, Fellows G. Bladder cancer after spinal cord injury. *Paraplegia* 1981;19: 265–70.

Frankel H, Mathias C. Cardiovascular aspects of autonomic dysreflexia since Guttmann and Whitteridge (1947). *Paraplegia* 1979;17:46–51.

Freed M, Bakst H, Barrie D. Life expectancy, survival rates, and causes of death in civilian patients with spinal cord trauma. *Arch Phys Med Rehabil* 1966;47:457–63.

Frisbie J, Kache A. Increasing survival and changing causes of death in myelopathy patients. *J Am Paraplegia Soc* 1983;6:51–6.

Geisler W, Jousse A, Wynne-Jones M. Survival in traumatic transverse myelitis. *Paraplegia* 1977;14:262–75.

Geisler W, Jousse A, Wynne-Jones M, Breithaupt D. Survival in traumatic spinal cord injury. *Paraplegia* 1983;21:364–73.

Gilliom JC. Personal communication, September 1985.

Goffman E. *Asylums.* Garden City, NY: Anchor Books, 1961.

Goldiamond I. Coping and adaptive behaviors of the disabled. In: Albrecht G, ed. *The sociology of physical disability and rehabilitation.* Pittsburgh: University of Pittsburgh Press, 1976:97–138.

Hackler R. A 25-year prospective mortality study in the spinal cord injured patient: comparison with the long-term living paraplegic. *J Urol* 1977;117:486–8.

Halstead L, Wiechers D, Rossi C. Late effects of poliomyelitis: a national survey. In: Halstead L, Wiechers D, eds. *Late effects of poliomyelitis.* Miami: Symposia Foundation, 1985:11–32.

Herbison G, Jaweed M, Ditunno J. Clinical management of the partially innervated muscle. In: Halstead L, Wiechers D, eds. *Late effects of poliomyelitis.* Miami: Symposia Foundation, 1985:171–80.

Hilfiker D. *Healing the wounds: a physician looks at his work.* New York: Pantheon Books, 1985.

Hilfiker D. A doctor's view of modern medicine. *New York Times Magazine,* February 23, 1986.

Howell T, Fullerton D, Harvey R, Klein M. Depression in spinal cord injury patients. *Paraplegia* 1981;19:284–8.

Kaufman J, Fam B, Jacobs S, Cabilondo F, Yalla S, Kane J, Rossier A. Bladder cancer and squamous metaplasia in spinal cord injury patients. *J Urol* 1977;118:967–71.

Kayser-Jones JS. *Old, alone, and neglected: care of the aged in Scotland and the United States.* Berkeley: University of California Press, 1981.

Le C, Price M. Survival from spinal cord injury. *J Chronic Dis* 1982;35:487–92.

Lewis I, Sheps C. *The sick citadel: the American academic medical center and the public interest.* Cambridge, MA: Oelgeschlager, Gun, and Hain, 1983.

Lynch J. *The broken heart: the medical consequences of loneliness.* New York: Basic Books, 1977.

Lynch J. *The language of the heart.* New York: Basic Books, 1985.

Maynard F. Differential diagnosis of pain and weakness in post polio patients. In: Halstead L, Wiechers D, eds. *Late effects of poliomyelitis.* Miami: Symposia Foundation, 1985:33–41.

Meshkinpour H, Vaziri N, Gordon S. Gastrointestinal pathology in patients with chronic renal failure associated with spinal cord injury. *Am J Gastroenterol* 1982;77: 562–4.

Mirahmadi M, Barton C, Vaziri N, Gordon S, Penera N. Nutritional evaluation of hemodialysis patients with and without spinal cord injury. *J Am Paraplegia Soc* 1983;6: 36–40.

Munro D. The rehabilitation of patients totally paralyzed below the waist, with special reference to making them ambulatory and capable of earning their own living: V. An end result of 445 cases. *N Engl J Med* 1954;250:4–14.

New York Times. Nursing costs force elderly to sue spouses. March 6, 1986.

New York Times. Biological aspects of the aging process. June 10, 1986.

Nuseibeh I, Burr R. Survival time in paraplegics with certain urinary complications. *Paraplegia* 1982;20:270–6.

Nyquist R, Bors E. Mortality and survival in traumatic myelopathy during nineteen years, from 1946 to 1965. *Paraplegia* 1967;5:22–48.

O'Brien G. Locus of control, previous occupation, and satisfaction with retirement. *Aust J Psychol* 1981;33:305–18.

Ohry A, Shemesh Y, Rozin R. Are chronic spinal cord injured patients (SCIP) prone to premature aging? *Med Hypotheses* 1983;11:467–9.

Paffembarger R, Hyde R, Wing A, Hsieh C. Physical activity, all-cause mortality, and longevity of college alumni. *N Engl J Med* 1986;314:605–13.

Pahl M, Vaziri N, Gordon S, Tuero S. Cardiovascular pathology in dialysis patients with spinal cord injury. *Artif Organs* 1983;7:416–9.

Richards J. Psychological adjustment to spinal cord injury during first year after discharge from the rehabilitation hospital. *Arch Phys Med Rehabil* 1986;67:362–5.

Rusley R. Do you believe in first class or supersaver medicine? *Med Economics* 1984;61: 99–102.

Schultz R, Decker S. Long term adjustment to physical disability: the role of social support, perceived control, and self blame. Unpublished manuscript, Portland State University, 1984.

Schultz R, Rau M. Social support throughout the life course. In: Cohen S, Syme S, eds. *Social support and health.* New York: Academic Press, 1985:129–49.

Schultz R, Wood D. Middle aged and elderly spinal cord injured persons: the support person's perspective. Unpublished manuscript, Portland State University, 1985.

Selye H. *The stress of life.* New York: McGraw-Hill Book Company, 1956 and 1976.

Starr P. *The social transformation of American medicine.* New York: Basic Books, 1982.

Stock D, Cole J. *Cooperative living: a cooperative self-support system for severely disabled young adults.* Final report RSA Grant No. 13-P-55487/6-01. Houston: Texas Institute for Rehabilitation and Research, 1977.

Swenson E. *The relationship between locus of control expectancy and successful rehabilitation of the spinal cord injured.* Doctoral Dissertation, Arizona State University, 1976.

Tomlinson B. Changes in spinal cord motor neurons of possible relevance to the late effects of poliomyelitis. In: Halstead L, Wiechers D, eds. *Late effects of poliomyelitis.* Miami: Symposia Foundation, 1985:57–70.

Trieschmann R. Coping with a disability: a sliding scale of goals. *Arch Phys Med Rehabil* 1974;55:556–60.

Trieschmann R. *Spinal cord injuries: the psychological, social, and vocational adjustment.* Elmsford, NY: Pergamon Press, 1980 (out of print; second edition, 1987, New York: Demos Publications).

Trieschmann R. The interpersonal costs of rehabilitation. *Paraplegia News* 1984a;38: 28–31.

Trieschmann R. Vocational rehabilitation: a psychological perspective. *Rehabil Lit* 1984b;45:345–8.

Vaziri N. Chronic hemodialysis in end stage renal disease associated with paraplegia. *Int J Artif Organs* 1984a;7:111–4.

Vaziri N. Long term haemodialysis in spinal cord injured patients. *Paraplegia* 1984b;22: 110–4.

Vaziri N, Byrne C, Mirahmadi M, Golji H, Nikakhtar B, Alday B, Gordon S. Hematologic features of chronic renal failure associated with spinal cord injury. *Artif Organs* 1982a;6:69–72.

Vaziri N, Cesario T, Mootoo K, Zeien L, Gordon S, Byrne C. Bacterial infection in patients with chronic renal failure: occurrence with spinal cord injury. *Arch Int Med* 1982b;142:1273–6.

Vaziri N, Gordon S, Nikakhtar B. Lipid abnormalities in chronic renal failure associated with spinal cord injury. *Paraplegia* 1982c;20:183–9.

Weil A. *Health and healing: understanding conventional and alternative medicine.* Boston: Houghton-Mifflin Company, 1983.

Wiechers D. Pathophysiology and late changes of the motor unit after poliomyelitis. In: Halstead L, Wiechers D, eds. *Late effects of poliomyelitis.* Miami: Symposia Foundation, 1985:91–4.

Wohl S. *The medical industrial complex.* New York: Harmony Books, 1984.

Young J, Burns P, Bowen A, McCutchen R. *Spinal cord injury statistics: experiences of the regional spinal cord injury systems.* Phoenix, AZ: Good Samaritan Medical Center, 1982.

Zubek J (ed). *Sensory deprivation: fifteen years of research.* New York: Appleton-Century-Crofts, 1969.

Zukav G. *The dancing wu li masters: an overview of the new physics.* Toronto: Bantam Books, 1979.

Subject Index

145